Clinical
Calculations

$$1 \text{ gr} = 60 \text{ mg}$$
$$15 \text{ gr} = 1 \text{ g} = 1000 \text{ mg}$$
$$1000 \text{ mcg } (\mu g) = 1 \text{ mg}$$
$$1 \text{ kg} = 2.2 \text{ lb}$$
$$1 \text{ mL } (1 \text{ cc}) = 15 \text{ ɱ}$$
$$4 \text{ mL } (4 \text{ cc}) = 1 \text{ dr } (\mathfrak{z})$$
$$5 \text{ mL } (5 \text{ cc}) = 1 \text{ tsp } (t)$$
$$30 \text{ mL } (30 \text{ cc}) = 1 \text{ oz } (\mathfrak{\tilde{z}}) = 2 \text{ tbs } (T) = 6 \text{ tsp } (t) = 8 \text{ dr } (\mathfrak{z})$$
$$500 \text{ mL } (500 \text{ cc}) = 1 \text{ pt } (0) = 16 \text{ oz } (\mathfrak{\tilde{z}})$$
$$1000 \text{ mL } (1000 \text{ cc}) = 1 \text{ L} = 1 \text{ qt} = 32 \text{ oz } (\mathfrak{\tilde{z}})$$

Clinical Calculations:
A Unified Approach
FOURTH EDITION

JOANNE M. DANIELS, RN, BSN, MSN
Professor Emeritus
SUNY College of Technology at Alfred, Alfred, NY

LORETTA M. SMITH, RN, BSN, MEd.
Professor Emeritus
SUNY College of Technology at Alfred, Alfred, NY

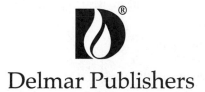

Delmar Publishers

an International Thomson Publishing company I(T)P®

Albany • Bonn • Boston • Cincinnati • Detroit • London • Madrid
Melbourne • Mexico City • New York • Pacific Grove • Paris • San Francisco
Singapore • Tokyo • Toronto • Washington

Notice to the Reader

Publisher does not warrant or guarantee any of the products described herein or perform any independent analysis in connection with any of the product information contained herein. Publisher does not assume, and expressly disclaims, any obligation to obtain and include information other than that provided to it by the manufacturer.

The reader is expressly warned to consider and adopt all safety precautions that might be indicated by the activities herein and to avoid all potential hazards. By following the instructions contained herein, the reader willingly assumes all risks in connection with such instructions.

The publisher makes no representation or warranties of any kind, including but not limited to, the warranties of fitness for particular purpose or merchantability, nor are any such representations implied with respect to the material set forth herein, and the publisher takes no responsibility with respect to such material. The publisher shall not be liable for any special, consequential, or exemplary damages resulting, in whole or part, from the readers' use of, or reliance upon, this material.

Delmar Staff

Publisher: *William Brottmiller*
Editor: *Greg Vis*
Production Coordinator: *Sandra Woods*
Art and Design Coordinator: *Jay Purcell*
Editorial Assistant: *Diane Biondi*
Cover Design: *Jay Purcell*

COPYRIGHT © 1999
By Delmar Publishers
an International Thomson Publishing Company, Inc.

The ITP logo is a trademark under license.

Printed in the United States of America

For more information, contact:

Delmar Publishers
3 Columbia Circle, Box 15015
Albany, New York 12212-5015

International Thomson Publishing Europe
Berkshire House
168-173 High Holborn
London, WC1V7AA
United Kingdom

Nelson ITP, Australia
102 Dodds Street
South Melbourne,
Victoria, 3205 Australia

Nelson Canada
1120 Birchmont Road
Scarborough, Ontario
M1K 5G4, Canada

International Thomson Publishing France
Tour Maine-Montparnasse
33 Avenue du Maine
75755 Paris Cedex 15, France

International Thomson Editores
Seneca 53
Colonia Polanco
11560 Mexico D. F. Mexico

International Thomson Publishing GmbH
Königswinterer Strasße 418
53227 Bonn
Germany

International Thomson Publishing Asia
60 Albert Street
#15-01 Albert Complex
Singapore 189969

International Thomson Publishing Japan
Hirakawa-cho Kyowa Building, 3F
2-2-1 Hirakawa-cho, Chiyoda-ku,
Tokyo 102, Japan

ITE Spain/ Paraninfo
Calle Magallanes, 25
28015-Madrid, Espana

2 3 4 5 6 7 8 9 10 XXX 02 01 00 99 98

Library of Congress Cataloging-in-Publication Data

Daniels, Joanne M.
    Clinical calculations : a unified approach / Joanne M. Daniels,
Loretta M. Smith. — 4th ed.
        p.   cm.
    Includes bibliographical references and index.
    ISBN 0-7668-0167-5
    1. Pharmaceutical arithmetic. 2. Drugs—Dosage.
    3. Drugs—Administration. 4. Nursing—Mathematics. I. Smith, Loretta M.
II. Title.
RS57.D36   1998
615'.14—dc21   98-15353
                                                  CIP

Contents

CHAPTER 10   **CALCULATIONS OF INTRAVENOUS MEDICATIONS AND SOLUTIONS   148**

CHAPTER 11   **ADMINISTRATION OF INTRAVENOUS MEDICATIONS AND SOLUTIONS   209**

CHAPTER 12   **PEDIATRIC DOSAGE   218**

CHAPTER 13   CLINICAL CALCULATIONS   236

Preface

Clinical Calculations offers students and practitioners alike the opportunity to develop skill in solving dosage problems using *dimensional analysis* (also known as the label factor method). This method is a logical and systematic approach to solving any type of medication administration problem. The method can be used with any system of measurement and facilitates conversion from one system to another. It easily replaces all other procedures for calculating medication dosages.

The advantages of a unified approach to clinical calculations include protection and precision, as well as ease and efficiency. The variety of approaches to dosage computations can be confusing and perplexing. A logical system is needed to significantly reduce errors made when medications are administered or dispensed. Dimensional analysis is such a system.

The text applies this versatile method to a cross section of computational applications typical of the clinical setting. These applications include calculating adult and pediatric oral and parenteral dosages, as well as intravenous flow rates and infusion times. Numerous solved examples guide the learner in using the method for these applications. Self-quizzes provide the opportunity for learners to practice dimensional analysis.

In the fourth edition, the methodology for application of dimensional analysis has been rewritten to simplify and amplify the process with additional examples and practice for each component step, making the process more user-friendly and better adapted to self-study. The name *label factor method,* which was used to identify the methodology in previous editions, has been replaced by dimensional analysis to correspond with the name more familiar to students who have previously learned the method in chemistry courses.

The text includes a detailed review of the routes by which medications are administered, particularly as they relate to the different types of dosage calculations. Performance criteria checklists for each route of administration provide a means of documenting learner progress in mastering the techniques.

The section on accountability has been amplified by the addition to practice problems of the question "Does my answer make sense?" Thus, students are encouraged to examine and analyze computational problems and answers in terms of common sense as well as memorized rules, to anticipate logical answers, and avoid medication errors.

This textbook is suitable for use in either traditional lecture classes, small group tutorial classes, or self-instruction. The fourth edition contributes to the self-instructional mode of learning. It provides more detailed explanations of dimensional analysis as it is used in different applications to help learners understand the method. To enhance practice in the reading of labels for identification of information essential to computations, 65 labels have been added making a total of 185 labels in the text. These labels familiarize learners with commonly prescribed drugs and provide opportunities for hands-on computation practice. All drugs have been updated and identified by generic names.

Ample space for working problems has been provided throughout the text making it usable as a workbook and helping to avoid errors in transcribing problems to a work sheet.

To the fourth edition has been added content on Celsius/Fahrenheit temperature conversions, fluid balance recording, computerized MAR and use of the twenty-four hour clock.

Content includes use of dimensional analysis for nutritional calculations and titration of infusions. Calculations applicable to critical care situations have been so identified.

Content   Chapter 1 introduces dimensional analysis, teaches the basic steps, and provides practice problems for each step as well as for the entire procedure.

Chapters 2–5 review the three systems of measurement (metric, apothecaries, and household) commonly used in prescribing medications and apply dimensional analysis to conversions within and between the systems.

Chapters 6 and 7 focus on medications administered by the oral route. Dimensional analysis is used in Chapter 6 to determine dosages of medications, both liquid and solid. In Chapter 7, general considerations related to safe and effective administration of oral medications and performance criteria are included, as are terms and abbreviations.

Chapters 8 and 9 apply dimensional analysis to dosage computations for medications administered parenterally (exclusive of intravenous administration), specifically via intradermal, subcutaneous, and intramuscular routes. General considerations, methodology, equipment, location of sites, and performance criteria are included in Chapter 9.

Chapters 10 and 11 focus on intravenous computations and administration. In Chapter 10 dimensional analysis is applied to the various computational problems associated with intravenous (IV) flow rate, infusion times, titrated medication additives, infusions, and parenteral nutrition. Chapter 11 describes the various routes of IV administration and includes sample problems and performance criteria.

Chapter 12 applies dimensional analysis to the calculation of pediatric dosages based on body weight or body surface area. Also included are general considerations related to administering medications to infants and children.

Chapter 13 summarizes the application of dimensional analysis. Two hundred twenty clinical problems offer a variety of examples of all of the preceding types of calculations. This unit can serve as a performance evaluation tool and a useful reference or review.

The appendix section of the text contains seven parts. Although it is assumed that learners using this text are familiar with elementary mathematics, Appendix A includes a variety of drill problems for review or practice in basic arithmetic processes. Students who require additional review or remediation are encouraged to seek the assistance of faculty or other sources.

Appendices B to E contain miscellaneous information which, although unrelated to dimensional analysis, is typically encountered in the clinical situation, including conversion between Celsius and Fahrenheit temperatures, measuring and recording fluid balance, dimensional analysis variation, and twenty-four hour clock.

Appendix F applies dimensional analysis to the calculation of components for the preparation of percentage solutions.

Finally, Appendix G contains the answers to all of the self-quizzes and problems in the text.

The text also includes an interactive CD ROM multimedia presentation that shows sample problems, review questions, and a testing component. The program provides scoring, helpful hints, animations, and color photos and illustrations. It is designed for individual, self-paced learning at home or in the comupter lab.

A valuable adjunct to the text for teachers looking for additional problems is an Instructor's Guide containing the answers to all quizzes and solutions to all practice problems, and a test bank of 100 problems with solutions. The Instructor's Guide also contains many useful and time-tested hints for effectively teaching the methodology. New features and teacher aids should make this edition particularly attractive to instructors.

Acknowledgments   We wish to express our sincere appreciation to the many individuals whose interest and assistance sustained and supported our efforts throughout the revision of this text.

We are especially grateful to our reviewers for their constructive and instructive critiques as well as their excellent ideas and suggestions, which have added new depth and dimension to the present edition.

Rick Berquist, RPh
Supervising Pharmacist
Eckerd Drugs
Hornell, New York

Susan Harrell, RN, MSN
Assistant Professor of Nursing
Dona Ana Branch Community College
Las Cruces, New Mexico

Cynthie Luehman, RN, MSN
Professor and Department of Nursing Chair
SUNY College of Technology at Alfred
Alfred, New York

Janice MacQuinn, RN-C, MSN
Assistant Professor of Nursing
South Georgia College
Douglas, Georgia

Judy Samsel, RN, MS
Associate Professor of Nursing
Broome Community College
Binghamton, New York

Lynn Stover, RN-C, MSN
Instructor
University of Alabama Capstone College of Nursing
Tuscaloosa, Alabama

Joanne Tate, RN, PhD
Teaching Specialist
Shadyside Hospital School of Nursing
Pittsburgh, Pennsylvania

Appreciation is expressed also to the following agencies and companies that supplied labels and photographs for illustrations and permission for use of copyrighted materials:

Abbott Laboratories, North Chicago, IL

Apothecon, Princeton, NJ

Arrow International, Inc., Reading, PA

Bard Med Systems Division, North Reading, PA

Baxter Healthcare Corporation, Deerfield, IL

Boehringer Ingelheim Pharmaceuticals, Inc., Ridgefield, CT

Bristol-Myers Squibb Co., Princeton, NJ

Bristol-Myers Squibb Oncology/Immunology Div., Princeton, NJ

Bristol-Myers Squibb U.S. Pharmaceutical Group, Evansville, IN

Critikon Inc., Tampa, FL

Dista Products Company, Division of Eli Lilly & Co., Indianapolis, IN

Eli Lilly and Company, Indianapolis, IN

Elkins-Sinn, Inc., Cherry Hill, NJ

Glaxo Wellcome, Inc., Research Triangle Park, NC

Hoechst Marion Roussel, Inc., Kansas City, MO

Hoffman LaRoche, Inc., Nutley, NJ

IVAC Corporation, San Diego, CA

Janssen Pharmaceutical, Inc., Piscataway, NJ

John C. Moore Corporation, Rochester, NY

Lederle Laboratories, Carolina, Puerto Rico

Lypho Med, Inc., Rosemont, IL

McNeil Pharmaceutical, Spring House, PA

Marsam Pharmaceuticals, Inc., Cherry Hill, NJ

Medical Information Technology Inc., Westwood, MA

Merck and Company Inc., West Point, PA

Mylan Pharmaceutical Inc., Morgantown, WV

Novartis Pharmaceutical Corporation, East Hanover, NJ

Novo Nordisk Pharmaceuticals Inc., Princeton, NJ

Pfizer Incorporated, New York, NY

Pharmacia and Upjohn Company, Kalamazoo, MI

Reed & Carnrick, Division of Block Drug Company, Inc., Jersey City, NJ

Rhone-Poulenc Rorer Pharmaceuticals Inc., Collegeville, PA

A.H. Robins Company, Inc., Richmond, VA

Roxane Laboratories, Inc., Columbus, OH

W. B. Saunders Company, Philadelphia, PA

Schering Corporation, Union, NJ

G. D. Searle & Co., Chicago, IL

SmithKline Beecham Pharmaceuticals, Philadelphia, PA

St. James Mercy Hospital, Hornell, NY

The Upjohn Company, Kalamazoo, MI

Warner Lambert Company, Morris Plains, NJ

Winthrop Breon Laboratories, Division of Sterling Drug, New York, NY

Wyeth-Ayerst Laboratories, Philadelphia, PA

Last, but surely not least, our loving thanks to Stu and Ang for fealty, fortitude, and forbearance above and beyond the call of husbandry.

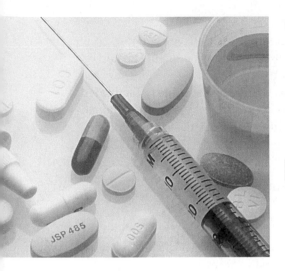

CHAPTER 1

Dimensional Analysis

OBJECTIVES

Upon completion of this chapter you should be able to:

- Analyze computation problems in order to identify the starting factor and the label for the answer.
- Analyze computation problems to identify equivalents given and equivalents needed.
- Set up an appropriate sequence of unit factors, called a conversion equation, whereby successive units can be cancelled.
- Correctly solve the conversion equation using cancellation and arithmetic to arrive at the answer in desired units.

This text presents a comprehensive approach to clinical calculations that is unique, uniform, and understandable. The term *clinical calculations* refers to the solving of computational problems associated with the administration of medications, specifically, determining the correct dosage to be given. Because these computations often involve converting from one system of measurement to another, it is essential that an accurate, reliable, and consistent method of solving conversion problems be utilized.

Introduction

Many drug and dose calculation textbooks dealing with mathematics relative to clinical practice use the methods of *ratio and proportion* and/or *desire over have times quantity* for the conversion of units of measure. Where two or more conversions are involved, these methods often become cumbersome and confusing to the learner. Frequently, the learner must remember a certain procedure or a different approach for each type of problem. This attempt to memorize several procedures involving similar units may be perplexing and discouraging.

We attempt to bring order out of confusion by using a consistent method, dimensional analysis, for all conversion problems.

Dimensional Analysis Methodology

Dimensional analysis, also known as label factor method or unit-conversion method, is a computation method whereby one particular unit of measurement is converted to another unit of measurement by use of a conversion factor or factors. This method focuses on the particular quantity of units in a problem that needs to be converted to equivalent units in another system of measurement. This known quantity and unit is called the starting factor. With consistent practice, the learner soon develops the ability to find this key item (starting factor). From this point on, equivalent values, called conversion factors, are utilized to convert from one system of units to another, leading, finally, to the desired unit (answer). These conversion factors fall into two categories that have either been (1) learned or (2) obtained from tables. With practice, conversion factors become very familiar and recognizable to the learner and, soon, this familiarity facilitates almost automatic application of the method to all conversion problems. Once the technique has been mastered, all other formulas or methodologies can be discarded.

Other advantages of dimensional analysis include:

- Eliminating memorization of different procedures and formulas for various types of problems.
- Enhancing the ability to analyze all problems in a systematic manner.
- Requiring only one equation and simple arithmetic, resulting in a very powerful mathematical tool that is almost foolproof.
- Applying the method to clinical calculation is both rapid and facile. Many students are already familiar with dimensional analysis because it is a computational technique taught in basic chemistry courses.

Dimensional Analysis

Definitions

1. Dimensional analysis is a computation method whereby one particular unit of measurement is converted to another unit of measurement by use of a conversion factor or factors.
2. A conversion factor is an equivalent value that can be used as a bridge between units of measurement without changing their value.

Steps in Dimensional Analysis

Dimensional analysis is composed of three steps:

1. Determining the starting factor and answer unit.
2. Formulating a conversion equation consisting of a sequence of labeled factors, in which successive units can be cancelled until the desired answer unit is reached.
3. Solving the conversion equation by use of cancellation and simple arithmetic.

Step I Determining the Starting Factor and Answer Unit

Initially, it is essential to determine exactly what information is sought. This information goal involves converting from one type of unit to another.

EXAMPLE   How many seconds are there in 5 minutes?

To answer this question, it is necessary to convert from minute units to seconds units. Therefore, the known quantity and its unit (5 min) which is to be converted is called the **starting factor.** The desired unit to which the starting factor will be converted is called the **answer unit.** These two items, the starting factor and the answer unit become, respectively, the first and the final items in the conversion equation. When the computation of the conversion equation has been completed, the two units of measurement (minute and seconds) will have an equivalent relationship.

The starting factors and answer units are identified in the following:

EXAMPLE   How many feet are there in 12 yards?

This example requires converting from yards to feet.

Starting Factor	Answer Unit
12 yds	ft

EXAMPLE   How many inches are there in 29 feet?

This example requires converting from feet to inches.

Starting Factor	Answer Unit
29 ft	in

EXAMPLE   How many ounces are there in 6 cups?

This example requires converting from cups to ounces.

Starting Factor	Answer Unit
6 cups	oz

Quantities can be expressed in a variety of units. For example, milk can be purchased by the pint, quart, or gallon. Thus, the same starting factor can have a variety of answer labels depending on the units asked for.

EXAMPLE   Find the number of milliliters in 4 quarts.

How many ounces are contained in 4 quarts?

Determine the number of cups in 4 quarts.

Calculate how many pints equal 4 quarts.

In each of these instances, an equivalent amount is sought for the quantity and unit, 4 quarts. Thus, 4 quarts is a known quantity and unit that must be converted to an equivalent unit to solve a problem or answer a question. In the above examples, the starting factor is always 4 quarts but the answer labels are milliliters, ounces, cups, and pints. Each of the four computations results in equivalent relationships.

The following questions and answers further identify starting factors and answer units:

1. If you went to the bank and obtained 325 dollars worth of quarters, how many quarters would you receive?

    Answer: 325 dollars is the known quantity and unit that must be converted to a desired unit (quarters). The starting factor, therefore, is 325 dollars and the answer unit is quarters and these two units will have an equivalent relationship.

2. You have 6 quarters but need dimes to use at the laundromat. How many dimes would you receive from 6 quarters?

    Answer: 6 quarters is the known quantity and unit that must be converted to a desired unit (dimes). The starting factor, therefore, is 6 quarters and the answer unit is dimes and these two units will have an equivalent relationship.

3. How many milliliters are contained in 1 teaspoon?

   Answer: 1 teaspoon is the known quantity and unit that must be converted to a desired unit (milliliters). The starting factor, therefore, is 1 teaspoon and the answer unit is milliliters and these two units will have an equivalent relationship.

4. What is the weight in kilograms of a child weighing 40 pounds?

   Answer: 40 pounds is a known quantity and unit that must be converted to a desired unit (kilograms). The starting factor, therefore, is 40 pounds and the answer unit is kilograms and these two units will have an equivalent relationship.

5. How many 10 grain tablets are needed to administer 1 gram of medication?

   Answer: 1 gram is the known quantity and unit that must be converted to a desired unit (tablets). The starting factor, therefore, is 1 gram and answer unit is tablets and these two units will have an equivalent relationship.

REMEMBER

The starting factor is always the first item in the conversion equation. The answer unit is always the final item in the equation. When the conversion equation is solved, it will be seen that the starting factor and the labeled answer have formed an equivalent relationship. See also Appendix D Dimensional Analysis Variation.

PRACTICE
Identifying the Starting Factor and Answer Unit

1. How many milligrams are there in 3 grains?

   Starting Factor   Answer Unit

   _____   _____

2. How many pounds are there in 5 kilograms?

   Starting Factor   Answer Unit

   _____   _____

3. How many tablets should the patient receive if the physician ordered 250 milligrams?

   Starting Factor   Answer Unit

   _____   _____

4. How many capsules should the patient receive if the ordered dose was 0.5 grams?

   Starting Factor   Answer Unit

   _____   _____

5. How many milliliters should be administered if the dose is 250 milligrams?

   Starting Factor   Answer Unit

   _____   _____

6. How many quarters are equal to 650 pennies?

   Starting Factor   Answer Unit

   _____   _____

PRACTICE
Identifying the *Starting Factor and Answer Unit*

7. How many nickels are equal to 9 dimes?

Starting Factor	Answer Unit
_____	_____

8. What is the length in inches of a toothpick that measures 5.08 cm in length?

Starting Factor	Answer Unit
_____	_____

9. A marathon race is 26.2 miles. This would be equal to _____ kilometers?

Starting Factor	Answer Unit
_____	_____

10. An automobile gets 30 miles/gal and gasoline cost $1.50/gal. What is the total cost of gasoline for a trip of 350 miles?

Starting Factor	Answer Unit
_____	_____

(**Note:** See Appendix G for answer key.)

Step II
Formulating the Conversion Equation

The second step in dimensional analysis is to set up a sequential series of equivalent values called *conversion factors,* which function as bridges leading from the starting factor to the desired unit (answer). This is the conversion equation. The conversion equation is written in a manner whereby successive units can be cancelled until the only unit remaining is the desired unit for the answer. It is essential that conversion factors contain only true (1:1) relationships; that is, the numerator and denominator of each factor must be of equivalent value. Multiplying a number by 1 does not change its value and multiplying by a fraction equal to 1 also leaves the value unchanged. A fraction is equal to 1 when the numerator is equivalent to the denominator.

For example: 60 sec = 1 min

Therefore, $\dfrac{60 \text{ sec}}{1 \text{ min}} = 1$

Similarly, $\dfrac{1 \text{ min}}{60 \text{ sec}} = 1$

It is important to note that conversion factors may be constant or variable relationships. Constant relationships are absolutes; they do not vary regardless of the context in which they are used. On the other hand, variable relationships do not necessarily remain constant, as illustrated in the following examples. Note that all the following equivalent values are 1:1 relationships and when written as conversion factors, the denominators and numerators can be interchanged.

Constant Relationships

EXAMPLE

Equivalent Value: 15 gr = 1 g

Conversion Factor: $\dfrac{15 \text{ gr}}{1 \text{ g}}$ or $\dfrac{1 \text{ g}}{15 \text{ gr}}$

EXAMPLE   Equivalent Value: 1 kg = 2.2 lb

Conversion Factor: $\dfrac{1\ kg}{2.2\ lb}$ or $\dfrac{2.2\ lb}{1\ kg}$

EXAMPLE   Equivalent Value: 1 tsp = 5 mL

Conversion Factor: $\dfrac{1\ tsp}{5\ mL}$ or $\dfrac{5\ mL}{1\ tsp}$

Variable Relationships

EXAMPLE   Equivalent Value: 350 mg = 1 tab

Conversion Factor: $\dfrac{350\ mg}{1\ tab}$ or $\dfrac{1\ tab}{350\ mg}$

EXAMPLE   Equivalent Value: 350 mg = 2.5 mL

Conversion Factor: $\dfrac{350\ mg}{2.5\ mL}$ or $\dfrac{2.5\ mL}{350\ mg}$

EXAMPLE   Equivalent Value: 350 mg = 1 tsp

Conversion Factor: $\dfrac{350\ mg}{1\ tsp}$ or $\dfrac{1\ tsp}{350\ mg}$

Approximate Equivalents

In setting up conversion factors, the learner either must know the equivalent relationships in various systems of measurement or have this information available for reference. Because it is frequently necessary to convert from one system of measurement to another in the same problem, the use of exact equivalents for corresponding units often results in large and cumbersome fractions or decimals that are very inconvenient in calculations and that may contribute to error. Therefore, certain approximations have been accepted widely and are in general use as equivalents for converting between systems. Table 1-1 lists approximate equivalents that are most frequently used in the calculation of medication dosages or solutions.

Approximate equivalents sometimes fall within a range, e.g., 60–65 mg = 1 gr, 4–5 mL = dr 1, 15–16 ɱ = 1 mL. In addition, the pint and quart equivalents are rounded from 480 mL to 500 mL and 960 mL to 1000 mL, respectively. For purposes of clinical calculations in this text, the numbers in Table 5-1 (Chapter 5) will be used.

Prior to formulating the conversion equation, the learner may find it helpful to list the equivalent values that will be used as conversion factors. These are the items that function as bridges leading from the starting factor to the desired unit (answer).

EXAMPLE   Find the number of yards in 1.5 miles

Equivalents: 1 yd = 36 in

1 yd = 3 ft

5280 ft = 1 mi

TABLE 1-1   **Approximate Equivalents**

$$1 \text{ gr} = 60 \text{ mg}$$
$$15 \text{ gr} = 1 \text{ g} = 1000 \text{ mg}$$
$$1000 \text{ mcg} (\mu g) = 1 \text{ mg}$$
$$1 \text{ kg} = 2.2 \text{ lb}$$
$$1 \text{ mL} (1 \text{ cc}) = 15 \text{ mL}$$
$$4 \text{ mL} (4 \text{ cc}) = 1 \text{ dr} (\text{з})$$
$$5 \text{ mL} (5 \text{ cc}) = 1 \text{ tsp} (t)$$
$$30 \text{ mL} (30 \text{ cc}) = 1 \text{ oz} (\text{з}) = 2 \text{ tbs} (T) = 6 \text{ tsp} (t) = 8 \text{ dr} (\text{з})$$
$$500 \text{ mL} (500 \text{ cc}) = 1 \text{ pt} (O) = 16 \text{ oz} (\text{з})$$
$$1000 \text{ mL} (1000 \text{ cc}) = 1 \text{ L} = 1 \text{ qt} = 32 \text{ oz} (\text{з})$$

Key to Abbreviations

gr = grain	mL = milliliter	L = liter
mg = milligram	cc = cubic centimeter	qt = quart
g = gram	dr (з) = dram	
kg = kilogram	tsp (t) = teaspoon	
lb = pound	oz (з) = ounce	
ɱ = minim	tbs (T) = tablespoon	
gtt = drop	pt (O) = pint	

These are *constant* relationships familiar to most students.

EXAMPLE

How many 10 gr tablets are needed to administer 1 gram of medication?

Equivalents: 10 gr = 1 tab

15 gr = 1 g

(**Note:** 10 gr = 1 tab is a *variable* relationship. Information regarding variable relationships is obtainable from drug labels, handbooks, inserts, pharmacists, etc. Note also that the problem contains both constant and variable equivalents.)

Identifying Equivalents

Using Table 1-1, list all the equivalents needed to solve the following problems.

EXAMPLE

How many 0.5 pint bottles can be filled by 4 quarts of solution?

Analysis of the question identifies 4 quarts as the starting factor and bottles as the answer label. Therefore, the equation involves going from 4 quarts to an equivalent number of bottles. The steps would include quarts to pints to bottles.

Equivalents: 1 qt = 2 pts, 1 bottle = 0.5 pt

EXAMPLE   Find the number of feet in 60 inches.
Equivalents: 12 in = 1 ft

EXAMPLE   How many miles would a runner complete in 1 hour if he runs the mile in 4 minutes?
Equivalents: 1 mi = 4 min, 60 min = 1 hr

EXAMPLE   Change 250 mg to g.
Equivalents: 1 g = 1000 mg

EXAMPLE   0.5 lb is equivalent to how many kg?
Equivalents: 2.2 lb = 1 kg

PRACTICE
Identifying Equivalents

1. How many feet are there in 12 yards?

   Equivalents:

2. How many inches are there in 29 feet?

   Equivalents:

3. How many quarters in $25.00?

   Equivalents:

4. How many nickels are equal to 9 dimes?

   Equivalents:

5. What is the length in inches of a toothpick that measures 5.08 cm in length?

   Equivalents:

6. How many milligrams are there in 3 grains?

   Equivalents:

7. How many pounds are there in 5 kilograms?

   Equivalents:

8. How many 0.5 gram tablets should the patient receive if the physician ordered 250 milligrams?

   Equivalents:

9. How many 250 milligram capsules should the patient receive if the ordered dose was 0.5 grams?

   Equivalents:

10. How many milliliters would be administered if the order was for 2 teaspoons?

    Equivalents:

Setting Up the Sequence of Conversion Factors

The conversion equation is formulated so that all unwanted units can be cancelled except the designated answer unit. Start with the known quantity and unit and apply the conversion factors as needed to get an answer in the desired unit. When the desired unit appears in the numerator, no more conversion factors are needed.

EXAMPLE   Find the number of minutes in 90 seconds.

Equivalents: 1 min = 60 sec

| Starting Factor | Conversion Factor | Answer Unit |

Conversion Equation:

$$90 \text{ sec} \quad \times \quad \frac{1 \text{ min}}{60 \text{ sec}} \quad = \underline{\quad} \text{ min}$$

As long as conversion factors are true 1:1 relationships that equal 1, adding conversion factors to the equation does not change the value of the answer.

EXAMPLE   Convert 60 seconds to hours.

Equivalents: 1 min = 60 sec, 60 min = 1 hr

Starting Factor   Conversion Factor   Answer Unit

Conversion Equation:

$$60 \text{ sec} \times \frac{1 \text{ min}}{60 \text{ sec}} \times \frac{1 \text{ hr}}{60 \text{ min}} = \underline{\quad} \text{ hr}$$

Thus, it can be seen that units can be logically and sequentially cancelled, greatly reducing the chance of error or omission. In solving the problem, each numerator unit cancels the immediately following denominator unit, so that all unwanted units are removed until the desired unit for the answer is reached. For instance, in the first example, all units are cancelled until the desired unit (min) is reached, ending the equation. This is the answer unit that was identified in Step I. Similarly, in the second example, all units are cancelled until the desired unit (hr) is reached, which was previously identified as the answer unit. The conversion equation is shown in Table 1-2.

TABLE 1-2   Conversion Equation

Conversion Factors

$$\text{Known Quantity and Unit} \times \frac{1}{1} \times \frac{1}{1} \times \frac{1}{1} \times \frac{1}{1} = \text{Answer (in desired unit)}$$
(Starting Factor)

Equivalent Relationship

Summary of Step II

EXAMPLE   Find the number of yards in 1.5 miles.

Equivalents: 1 mi = 5280 ft; 3 ft = 1 yd

Starting Factor   Conversion Factors   Answer Unit

$$1.5 \text{ mi} \times \qquad \frac{5280 \text{ ft}}{1 \text{ mi}} \times \frac{1 \text{ yd}}{3 \text{ ft}} \qquad = \underline{\hspace{1cm}} \text{ yd}$$

The following observations regarding this problem summarize Step II of dimensional analysis.

- The starting factor is 1.5 mi, because this is the known quantity and unit that must be converted to an equivalent unit.

- In the two conversion factors, the units mile and feet are placed in the denominators to cancel the corresponding units of the immediately preceding factors. (*Note:* Make it a cardinal rule that each factor cancels a unit in the preceding factor.)

- The two conversion factors, 5280 ft/mi and 1 yd/3 ft are each equivalent relationships. That is, these factors have 1:1 value and do not change the actual value of the starting factor. Their purpose is to lead to an equivalent answer expressed in some other unit. The relationships in each factor must be true for the answer to be correct.

- The answer unit always appears in the numerator farthest to the right in the conversion equation (in the example above: yd).

REMEMBER

It is desirable that conversion factors be arranged in a sequence so that identical units are placed diagonally; that is, whatever unit appears in the numerator of one factor appears in the denominator of the factor immediately following.

Setting Up Conversion Equations

EXAMPLE   How many milligrams are there in 3 grains?

Equivalents: 60 mg = gr 1

Conversion Equation: $\cancel{\text{gr}} \, 3 \times \dfrac{60 \text{ mg}}{\cancel{\text{gr}} \, 1} = \underline{\hspace{1cm}} \text{ mg}$

EXAMPLE   How many pounds are there in 5 kilograms?

Equivalents: 1 kg = 2.2 lb

Conversion Equation: $5 \, \cancel{\text{kg}} \times \dfrac{2.2 \text{ lb}}{1 \, \cancel{\text{kg}}} = \underline{\hspace{1cm}} \text{ lb}$

EXAMPLE   How many tablets should the patient receive if the physician ordered 250 mg and each tablet contains 100 mg?

Equivalents: 1 tab = 100 mg

Conversion Equation: $250 \text{ mg} \times \dfrac{1 \text{ tab}}{100 \text{ mg}} = $ _____ tab

EXAMPLE   How many capsules should be administered if the order states gr 2 and the medication label states 60 mg/capsule?

Equivalents: gr 1 = 60 mg, 60 mg = 1 cap

Conversion Equation:

$$\text{gr } 2 \times \dfrac{60 \text{ mg}}{\text{gr } 1} \times \dfrac{1 \text{ cap}}{60 \text{ mg}} = \underline{\qquad} \text{ cap}$$

EXAMPLE   Change 5 grains to grams.

Equivalents: 15 gr = 1 g

Conversion Equation: $5 \text{ gr} \times \dfrac{1 \text{ g}}{15 \text{ gr}} = $ _____ g

Note that the last equation shows the most direct route from grains to grams. However, it can be seen from Table 1-1 that other equivalent relationships exist between grains and grams.

EXAMPLE   Equivalents: 15 gr = 1000 mg, 1000 mg = 1 g

Conversion Equation:

$$5 \text{ gr} \times \dfrac{1000 \text{ mg}}{15 \text{ gr}} \times \dfrac{1 \text{ g}}{1000 \text{ mg}} = \underline{\qquad} \text{ g}$$

EXAMPLE   Equivalents: 1 gr = 60 mg, 1000 mg = 1 g

Conversion Equation:

$$5 \text{ gr} \times \dfrac{60 \text{ mg}}{1 \text{ gr}} \times \dfrac{1 \text{ g}}{1000 \text{ mg}} = \underline{\qquad} \text{ g}$$

Thus, there may be several routes leading from one starting factor to an equivalent end value. Insofar as possible, it is best to choose the most direct route (i.e., that which requires the fewest conversion factors). Because many of the equivalent relationships, as pointed out before, are *approximations,* the use of additional conversion factors may result in small differences in the end result values. *Therefore, in some instances, the learner may obtain a slightly different answer from the answer key in Appendix G.* Some multiple answers have been included in the key but, obviously, others are possible. When a discrepancy is found, the learner should recheck for accuracy of arithmetic and equivalents. If these are correct, the alternative answer is acceptable. When there is a question as to a safe margin for accuracy, a pharmacist or a drug reference manual should be consulted. In any case, no more than a 10% difference should occur between the ordered dose of a medication and the amount administered.

PRACTICE
Setting Up Conversion Equations

1. How many mL should be administered if the dose is 250 mg and the label states 500 mg/tsp?

   Equivalents:

   Conversion Equation:

2. How many milliliters should the patient receive if the order states 125 mg and the medication strength is 250 mg/5 mL?

   Equivalents:

   Conversion Equation:

3. How many milliliters are necessary to follow the order of 0.75 g if the medication label states 0.5 g/ʒ 1?

   Equivalents:

   Conversion Equation:

4. How many tablets (scored) will be administered if the ordered dose is gr ⅛ and the tablet strength is 15 mg/tab?

   Equivalents:

   Conversion Equation:

5. How many milligrams would the patient receive if the order is for 15 mL and the medication strength is 300 mg/tsp?

   Equivalents:

   Conversion Equation:

6. What is the length in feet of a sofa that measures 84 inches?

   Equivalents:

   Conversion Equation:

7. A newborn weighs 6.5 lb at birth. What is his weight in kilograms?

   Equivalents:

   Conversion Equation:

9. How many milliliters are there in a 2.5 L bottle of soda pop?

   Equivalents:

   Conversion Equation:

8. A recipe calls for 675 mL of milk. How many ounces of milk will you need?

   Equivalents:

   Conversion Equation:

10. If a physician ordered 10 mL of a cough medicine, how many tsp should be administered?

    Equivalents:

    Conversion Equation:

(**Note:** See Appendix G for answer key.)

Step III
Solving the
Conversion Equation

The third step in dimensional analysis involves the use of cancellation and simple arithmetic to solve the equation formulated in Step II. Cancellation of labels, reduction of numerical values, and simple multiplication are used to solve the conversion equation.

$$5 \text{ min} \times \frac{60 \text{ sec}}{1 \text{ min}} = 300 \text{ sec}$$

Note that the known quantity and unit (starting factor), 5 min, and answer in desired units (answer label), 300 sec, have now formed an equivalent relationship; that is, 5 minutes has been converted to 300 seconds. Thus, dimensional analysis has been applied to convert one particular unit of measurement to another unit of measurement without changing the values.

If the series of conversion factors has been set up so that corresponding units are in sequential numerator/denominator positions, the numerical values can likewise be cancelled or reduced to lowest terms and appropriately multiplied to solve the equation. The resulting answer should be reduced to lowest terms, converted to a decimal, and/or rounded off, as appropriate.

Solving the Conversion Equation

EXAMPLE   How many tablets should be administered?

Order: Codeine 60 mg

Label: Codeine gr ½ per tab

Equivalents: 60 mg = gr 1, gr ½ = 1 tab

Conversion Equation: $60 \text{ mg} \times \dfrac{\text{gr } 1}{60 \text{ mg}} \times \dfrac{1 \text{ tab}}{\text{gr } \frac{1}{2}} = 2 \text{ tab}$

Does this answer make sense? Note the equivalent 60 mg = gr 1 and 1 tab = gr ½. If the order is for 60 mg it is obvious that more than 1 tablet is required. Therefore, an answer of less than 1 tablet should be recognized as incorrect.

EXAMPLE   How many milliliters should be administered?

Order: Vistaril 25 mg

Label: Vistaril (hydroxyzine HCl) 100 mg/2 mL

Equivalents: 100 mg = 2 mL

Conversion Equation: $25 \text{ mg} \times \dfrac{2 \text{ mL}}{100 \text{ mg}} = 0.5 \text{ mL}$

Does this answer make sense? Note the equivalent 100 mg = 2 mL. If the order is for 25 mg, it is obvious that less than 2 mL is required. Therefore, an answer of 2 mL more would not make sense.

EXAMPLE   How many 0.5 pint bottles can be filled by 4 quarts of solution?

Equivalents: 1 qt = 2 pt, 1 bottle = 0.5 pt

Conversion Equation: $4 \text{ qt} \times \dfrac{2 \text{ pt}}{1 \text{ qt}} \times \dfrac{1 \text{ bottle}}{0.5 \text{ pt}} = 16 \text{ bottles}$

Does this answer make sense? It can be seen that a bottle is a much smaller container than a quart. Therefore, the number of bottles in the answer must be larger than the number of quarts.

EXAMPLE   Change 250 mg to g.

Equivalents: 1 g = 1000 mg

Conversion Equation: $250 \text{ mg} \times \dfrac{1 \text{ g}}{1000 \text{ mg}} = 0.25 \text{ g}$

Does this answer make sense? If it takes 1000 mg to make 1 g, it makes sense to expect that 250 mg would be less than 1 g.

EXAMPLE   What is the equivalent in kilograms of 0.5 lb?

Equivalents: 2.2 lb = 1 kg

Conversion Equation: $0.5 \, \cancel{lb} \times \dfrac{1 \text{ kg}}{2.2 \, \cancel{lb}} = 0.23 \text{ kg}$

Does this answer make sense? If 1 kg is equivalent to 2.2 lb, it is obvious that 0.5 lb would be far less than 1 kg.

(**Note:** Refer to Appendix A for basic arithmetic review.)

The learner who is having difficulty solving equations should seek remedial assistance before proceeding further.

REMEMBER

1. Be sure the starting factor is the first item and the answer unit is the last item in the conversion equation.
2. Use only conversion factors that have a 1:1 relationship.
3. Set up the conversion equation so that cancellable units appear in consecutive numerator/denominator.
4. When solving the conversion equation:

   - cancel units first.
   - reduce numbers to lowest terms.
   - multiply/divide to solve the equation.
   - reduce answer to lowest terms, convert to decimal, and/or round off.

5. Always think about whether your answer makes sense.

PRACTICE
Solving Conversion Equations

1. **Order:** Lanoxin 0.250 mg
   Label: Lanoxin (digoxin) 0.125 mg/tab

   Question: How many tablets should the patient receive? _____

   Equivalents:

   Conversion Equation:

   Does your answer make sense?

2. **Order:** Nembutal gr ½
   Label: Nembutal (pentobarbital) 30 mg/cap

   Question: How many capsules should the nurse give? _____

   Equivalents:

   Conversion Equation:

   Does your answer make sense?

PRACTICE
Solving Conversion Equations

3. **Order:** Tolinase 250 mg
   Label: Tolinase (tolazamide) 0.5 g/tab (scored)

   Question: How many tablets should be administered? _____

   Equivalents:

   Conversion Equation:

   Does your answer make sense?

4. **Order:** Morphine sulfate gr $\frac{1}{6}$
   Label: Morphine sulfate gr $\frac{1}{4}$ per 1.4 mL

   Question: How many mL should be administered? _____

   Equivalents:

   Conversion Equation:

   Does your answer make sense?

5. **Order:** Atropine sulfate gr $\frac{1}{100}$
   Label: Atropine sulfate gr $\frac{1}{150}$ per mL

   Question: How many mL should be administered? _____

Equivalents:

Conversion Equation:

Does your answer make sense?

6. **Order:** Chloral hydrate elixir 1 g
   Label: Chloral hydrate elixir gr 7 $\frac{1}{2}$ per 5 mL

   Question: How many mL will equal this dose? _____

   Equivalents:

   Conversion Equation:

   Does your answer make sense?

7. **Order:** Riopan 10 mL
   Label: Riopan (magaldrate) 400 mg/tsp

   Question: How many mg will be contained in this dose? _____

   Equivalents:

   Conversion Equation:

   Does your answer make sense?

PRACTICE
Solving Conversion Equations

8. **Order:** Ceclor 200 mg
   Label: Ceclor (cefaclor) 125 mg/5 mL

   Question: How many mL must be
   administered? _____

   Equivalents:

   Conversion Equation:

   Does your answer make sense?

9. **Order:** Dilantin 30 Pediatric Suspension 75 mg
   Label: Dilantin 30 (phenytoin sodium)
   Pediatric Suspension 30 mg/5 mL

   Question: How many mL should be
   administered? _____

Equivalents:

Conversion Equation:

Does your answer make sense?

10. **Order:** Phenobarbital 90 mg
    Label: Phenobarbital gr 1 ½ per tab

    Question: How many tablets should be
    given? _____

    Equivalents:

    Conversion Equation:

    Does your answer make sense?

(**Note:** See Appendix G for answer key.)

**Accuracy and
Accountability**

The learner is cautioned against blind reliance on any formula, particularly when its use has become familiar and automatic. The application of common sense and reasonable prudence will help prevent medication errors due to either carelessness or inaccuracy in determining equivalents and solving conversion equations.

Although the level of arithmetic required to solve nearly all dimensional analysis problems is almost elementary, math errors do occur. This means that it is essential to double-check the computation, even if a calculator is used.

To this end, the learner should develop the habit of carefully inspecting the information given in every problem and seeking simple benchmarks relative to the anticipated answer. For example, should it be less than or more than one tablet, grain, or milliliter? What is a typical and reasonable amount of solution for an intravenous, an intramuscular, or an oral medication? Extremely large numbers should be suspect: answers such as 12 tablets po, 850 gtt/min IV, 16 mL IM should be questioned as *illogical* and *unreasonable*. When there is any doubt as to the accuracy of a computation, a drug reference should be consulted to be sure the answer is consistent with the recommended range of dosage for that particular drug. An additional resource for verification is the registered pharmacist.

Medication errors constitute one of the greatest areas of risk for which health-care providers can be vulnerable to negligence or malpractice litigation. Although it is hoped that the use of a single and consistent approach to calculating medication dosages will help prevent medication errors, it must be emphasized that any method or formula is only as safe as the individual using it.

REMEMBER

The final step in solving any problem, of course, is to ask whether the answer is reasonable. Common sense and common caution are prerequisites for using dimensional analysis in clinical calculations.

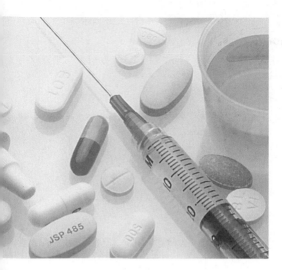

CHAPTER 2

The Metric System of Measurement

Upon completion of this chapter you should be able to:

- Identify the three basic units of measurement in the metric system: gram, liter, and meter.
- List metric abbreviations and prefixes commonly used in drug computations.
- Compare various metric units in relation to length, weight, and volume.
- Apply dimensional analysis to conversions within the metric system.

Basic Units

The basic units of measurement in the metric system are the gram as the unit of weight, the liter as the unit of volume, and the meter as the unit of length. These basic units can be divided or multiplied into various related units as seen in Table 2-1. The main feature of the metric system is that each of the basic units may be divided into decimal values or expanded into multiples of ten by the use of standard prefixes, Table 2-2.

Comparing Metric Units

When converting metric values, make use of the obvious principle: "It takes many small units to equal a large unit." For example, in Table 2-3, it can be seen that a milligram is 0.001 gram and is a small unit. It would take 1000 milligrams to equal one gram, Figure 2-1. However, a kilogram is a large unit. It takes 1000 grams to equal one kilogram. Similarly, a milliliter is 0.001 L and is a small unit, Table 2-4. It takes 1000 mL to equal one liter, Figure 2-2. Finally, the small unit, millimeter, equals one one thousandth of a meter, Table 2-5. It takes 10 millimeters to equal 1 centimeter and 100 centimeters to equal 1 meter, Figure 2-3.

Obviously, there are many more divisions and multiples of the basic metric units possible. Tables 2-1 to 2-5 contain the quantities most frequently used in clinical calculations of dosages and measurements; these relationships should be memorized.

Metric Notation

In the metric system, quantities are written with the number preceding the unit. Arabic whole numbers and decimals are used rather than Roman numerals or fractions. See examples in Table 2-6.

TABLE 2-1   Metric Units and Abbreviations

Unit	Abbreviations
weight	
gram	g
milligram	mg
microgram*	mcg
kilogram	kg
volume	
liter	L
milliliter**	mL
minim	ꝳ
length	
meter	m
centimeter	cm
millimeter	mm

*The symbol μg is often used on a drug label as an abbreviation for microgram
**A milliliter is a small unit of volume frequently used in dispensing medication. It has the same volume as a cubic centimeter (cc). The abbreviations cc and mL may be used interchangeably.

TABLE 2-2   Metric Prefixes

Small Units	Large Units
deci = 0.1	deka = 10
centi = 0.01	hecto = 100
milli = 0.001	kilo = 1,000
micro = 0.000001	mega = 1,000,000

TABLE 2-3   Metric Units of Weight

Many Small Units Equal One Large Unit
1 mg = 0.001 g; 1000 mg = 1 g
1 mcg (μg) = 0.000001 g; 1,000,000 mcg (μg) = 1 g
1 mcg (μg) = 0.000001 g; 1000 mcg (μg) = 1 mg
1 g = 0.001 kg; 1000 g = 1 kg

TABLE 2-4   Metric Units of Volume

Many Small Units Equal One Large Unit
1 mL (1 cc) = 0.001 L; 1000 mL = 1 L

TABLE 2-5   *Metric Units of Length*

Many Small Units Equal One Large Unit
1 mm = 0.001 m; 1000 mm = 1 m
1 cm = 0.01 m; 100 cm = 1 m

TABLE 2-6   **Metric Notation**

Quantity	Notation
1 gram	1 g
60 milligrams	60 mg
3 liters	3 L
500 milliliters	500 mL
10 meters	10 m
150 centimeters	150 cm

FIGURE 2-1
Weight (metric)

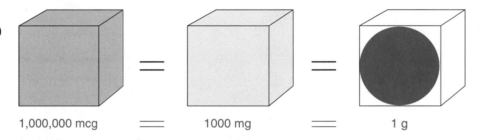

1,000,000 mcg = 1000 mg = 1 g

FIGURE 2-2
Volume (metric)

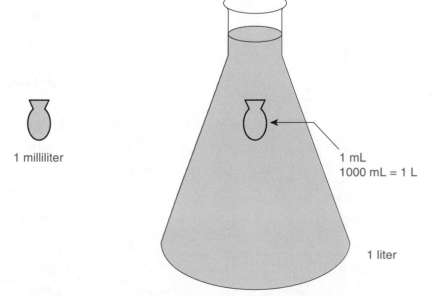

1 milliliter

1 mL
1000 mL = 1 L

1 liter

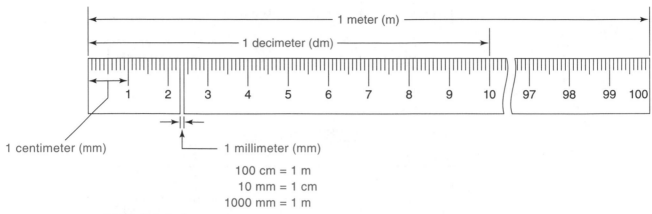

100 cm = 1 m
10 mm = 1 cm
1000 mm = 1 m

FIGURE 2-3
Length (metric)

Converting Units within the Metric System

Using the previously memorized prefixes and relationships as equivalent values, complete the practice problems following the steps used in examples a–d. (Carry each answer to two decimal places and round to nearest tenth.)

EXAMPLE

Convert 0.16 centimeters to millimeters.

Starting Factor	Answer Unit
0.16 cm	mm

Equivalents: 1 cm = 0.01 m; 1 mm = 0.001 m

Conversion Equation:

$$0.16 \text{ cm} \times \frac{0.01 \text{ m}}{1 \text{ cm}} \times \frac{1 \text{ mm}}{0.001 \text{ m}} = 1.6 \text{ mm}$$

EXAMPLE

Convert 240 micrograms to milligrams.

Starting Factor	Answer Unit
240 mcg	mg

Equivalents: 1 mg = 1000 mcg

Conversion Equation:

$$240 \text{ mcg} \times \frac{1 \text{ mg}}{1000 \text{ mcg}} = 0.2 \text{ mg}$$

EXAMPLE

Convert 375 milligrams to grams.

Equivalents: 1000 mg = 1 g; 1 mg = 0.001 g

Conversion Equation:

$$375 \text{ mg} \times \frac{1 \text{ g}}{1000 \text{ mg}} = 0.4 \text{ g}$$

OR

$$375 \text{ mg} \times \frac{0.001 \text{ g}}{1 \text{ mg}} = 0.4 \text{ g}$$

EXAMPLE   Convert 75 grams to kilograms.

Equivalents: 1000 g = 1 kg; 1 g = 0.001 kg

Conversion Equation:

$$75\,g \times \frac{1\,kg}{1000\,g} = 0.1\,kg$$

OR

$$75\,g \times \frac{0.001\,kg}{1\,g} = 0.1\,kg$$

PRACTICE
Convert within the Metric System

1. 3225 mL to L

6. 0.75 L to mL

2. 375 mg to g

7. 0.22 g to mg

3. 2000 g to kg

8. 2.5 kg to g

4. 5000 mcg to mg

9. 25 mm to cm

5. 29 cm to m

10. 12 mg to mcg

(**Note:** See Appendix G for answer key.)

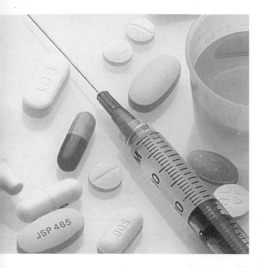

CHAPTER 3

The Apothecaries System of Measurement

OBJECTIVES

Upon completion of this chapter you should be able to:

- Identify the four basic units of measurement in the apothecaries system: grain, minim, fluid dram, fluid ounce.
- List apothecaries abbreviations and symbols commonly used in drug computations.
- Compare various apothecaries units in relation to weight and volume.
- Apply dimensional analysis to conversions within the apothecaries system.

Although the apothecaries system of measurement is being replaced by the metric, the former system is still sometimes used in writing prescriptions and medication orders. Therefore, the nurse should be familiar with it, particularly its symbols and abbreviations, Table 3-1.

Basic Units and Abbreviations

In the apothecaries system, the grain is the basic unit of weight and the minim, fluid dram, and fluid ounce are the basic units of volume. The latter two usually are shortened to dram and ounce. Although dry weights can be measured in drams and ounces, they are rarely so measured for medication computations. Therefore, when the terms dram and ounce are used in medication orders or calculations in this text, they refer to fluid volume. An exception to this rule is in the preparation of percentage solutions, which is illustrated in Appendix F. Additionally, the pint and quart are units of volume that are rarely used in the administration of medications.

When body weight is required for calculation of dosage, the pound unit is used. In the traditional apothecaries system, the pound consists of 12 (dry weight) ounces; however, it is common practice in this country to employ the 16 ounce avoirdupois pound for dry weights. Therefore, any computation involving conversions of pound units in this text "implies" use of the 16 ounce pound.

It is important to note the difference between the dram and ounce symbols, as seen in Table 3-1. The dram, which is a smaller amount, has one less loop than the ounce symbol, which represents the larger amount. **Confusion of these two symbols can result in a serious medication error.**

TABLE 3-1   *Basic Apothecaries Units*

Unit	Abbreviation
weight	
grain	gr
pound (16 oz)	lb
volume	
minim	♏
dram	dr or ℥
ounce	oz or ℥
pint	
pt or 0	
quarter	qt

Apothecaries Notation

When writing quantities in the apothecaries system, the number *follows* the unit, in contrast to the metric system. For small numbers up to 10, lower-case Roman numerals are used with a line drawn over the digits and a dot over each i. For numbers larger than 10, Arabic numbers may be substituted except for 20 (XX) and 30 (XXX).

Table 3-2 shows examples of traditional apothecaries notations. However, in the clinical setting, the practitioner frequently will encounter apothecaries notations written in the metric form, that is, Arabic numbers preceding the unit. The learner should become familiar with both methods of apothecaries notations; they are used interchangeably in this text.

Note, in particular, the use of the abbreviation s̄s. Used alone, this symbol means ½; when larger quantities are denoted: 1 ½, 2 ½, the appropriate numeral is placed to the left of the symbol.

Comparing Apothecaries Units

In comparing apothecaries values, the learner should keep in mind, as with metric units, that many small units equal one large unit. For example, a minim is a small amount; it takes 60 minims to equal one dram, Figure 3-1. However, a quart is a large unit; it would take 256 drams to equal one quart, Table 3-3.

TABLE 3-2   *Apothecaries Notation*

Quantity	Notation
⅒ grain	gr ⅒
1 grain	gr i
1 ½ grains	gr iss
10 grains	gr x
15 minims	♏ 15
150 minims	♏ 150
2 ½ ounces	℥ iiss

FIGURE 3-1
Liquid relationships
(apothecaries)

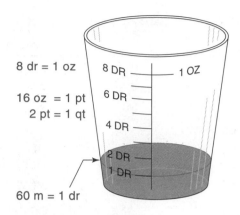

8 dr = 1 oz

16 oz = 1 pt
2 pt = 1 qt

60 m = 1 dr

PRACTICE
Write the abbreviation for each of the following

1. dram (symbol) = _____

2. grain = _____

3. minim = _____

4. one half = _____

5. ounce (symbol) = _____

(**Note:** See Appendix G for answer key.)

Converting Units within the Apothecaries System

Using the apothecaries equivalents, complete the practice problems following the steps used in the examples.

EXAMPLE Convert 30 minims to drams.

Starting Factor Answer Unit
30 m dr

Equivalents: 60 m = 1 dr

Conversion Equation: $30 \; \cancel{m} \times \dfrac{1 \; dr}{60 \; \cancel{m}} = \tfrac{1}{2} \; dr$

TABLE 3-3 *Apothecaries Fluid Units*

60 m = 1 dr (ʒ)
8 dr = 1 oz (℥)
16 oz = 1 pt (0)
2 pt = 1 qt

EXAMPLE　　Convert 64 drams to pints.

Starting Factor　　Answer Unit
64 dr　　　　　　　　pt

Equivalents: 8 dr = 1 oz, 16 oz = 1 pt

Conversion Equation:

$$64 \text{ dr} \times \frac{1 \text{ oz}}{8 \text{ dr}} \times \frac{1 \text{ pt}}{16 \text{ oz}} = \frac{1}{2} \text{ pt}$$

EXAMPLE　　Convert 55 ounces to quarts.

Starting Factor　　Answer Unit
55 oz　　　　　　　　qt

Equivalents: 32 oz = 1 qt

Conversion Equation:　$55 \text{ oz} \times \frac{1 \text{ qt}}{32 \text{ oz}} = 1 \frac{7}{10} \text{ qt}$

EXAMPLE　　Convert 4 drams to ounces.

Starting Factor　　Answer Unit
4 dr　　　　　　　　　oz

Equivalents: 8 dr = 1 oz

Conversion Equation:　$4 \text{ dr} \times \frac{1 \text{ oz}}{8 \text{ dr}} = \frac{1}{2} \text{ oz}$

EXAMPLE　　Convert pints iss to ʒ .

Starting Factor　　Answer Unit
1 ½ pt　　　　　　　oz

Equivalents: 1 pt = 16 oz, 1 oz = 8 dr

Conversion Equation:

$$1 \frac{1}{2} \text{ pt} \times \frac{16 \text{ oz}}{1 \text{ pt}} \times \frac{8 \text{ dr}}{1 \text{ oz}} = 192 \text{ dr}$$

PRACTICE
Convert within the Apothecaries System

1. 55 oz to qt

2. 4 dr to oz

3. pt iss to ℥

4. 30 ♏ to ℥

5. 2 mL to ℥

6. 1 ¼ oz to ʒ

7. 120 ♏ to ℥

8. 2 pts to dr

9. 3 ½ lb to oz

10. 62.4 oz to lb

(**Note:** See Appendix G for answer key.)

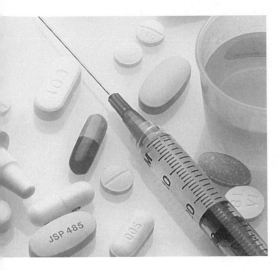

CHAPTER 4

The Household System of Measurement

OBJECTIVES

Upon completion of this chapter you should be able to:

- Identify the units of measurement in the household system: drops, teaspoons, tablespoons, cups, and glasses.
- List household abbreviations commonly used in drug computations.
- Compare various household units in relation to volume.
- Apply dimensional analysis to conversions within the household system.

Household Units

The household system of measurement involves the use of drops, spoons, cups, and glasses, Table 4-1. These units, which are derived from household measuring utensils, are not very precise. For example, the size of a drop of fluid will vary depending on the temperature, the composition of the fluid, and the size of the opening from which the drop emerges. The use of cups and spoons as measuring apparatus cannot compare to the accuracy of graduates and syringes as used with the metric system.

Household units are used primarily in the administration of external preparations such as baths, soaks, gargles, enemas, compresses, and disinfectants. They also are used in measuring oral fluid intake where a high

TABLE 4-1   Household Units

Unit	Abbreviation
volume	
drop	gtt
teaspoon	tsp or t
tablespoon	tbs or T
cup/glass	c/gl
pint	pt
quart	qt
gallon	gal
length	
inch	in
foot	ft

TABLE 4-2   Household Equivalents

60 gtt = 1 tsp
3 tsp = 1 tbs
2 tbs = 1 oz
6 oz = 1 teacup
8 oz = 1 glass or measuring cup
16 oz = 1 pt
2 pt = 1 qt
4 qt = 1 gal

degree of accuracy is not necessary. These units and their approximate equivalents are listed in Table 4-2.

The more commonly used units should be memorized, because of their frequency of use in the situations mentioned previously.

Household Notation   In the household system, quantities are written in the same manner as in the metric system; the number (quantity) precedes the unit and Arabic whole numbers are used. Fractions or decimals may be used for quantities that are portions of whole numbers, Table 4-3.

PRACTICE
Write the abbreviations for each of the following

1. drop   = _____

2. gallon   = _____

3. pint   = _____

4. tablespoon   = _____

5. teaspoon   = _____

(**Note:** See Appendix G for answer key.)

TABLE 4-3   Household Notation

Quantity	Notation
1 drop	1 gtt
3 teaspoons	3 tsp
8 ounces	8 oz
2 pints	2 pt

FIGURE 4-1
Liquid relationships (household)

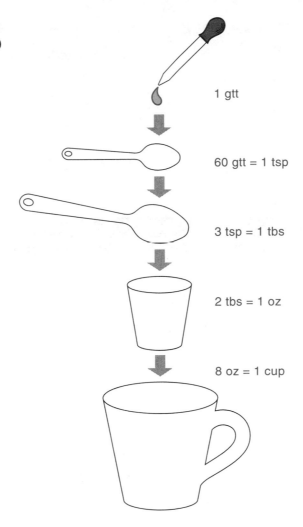

FIGURE 4-1
Liquid relationships (household)

1 gtt

60 gtt = 1 tsp

3 tsp = 1 tbs

2 tbs = 1 oz

8 oz = 1 cup

Comparing Household Units

Figure 4-1 illustrates the progression of the various units of volume in the household system of measurement.

Converting Units within the Household System

Using the relationships given as equivalent values, complete the practice problems following the steps used in the examples. (Carry each answer to two decimal places and round to nearest tenth.)

EXAMPLE

Convert 16 tablespoons to cups.

Starting Factor   Answer Unit
16 tbs   cup

Equivalents: 2 tbs = 1 oz; 8 oz = 1 cup

Conversion Equation:

$$16 \text{ tbs} \times \frac{1 \text{ oz}}{2 \text{ tbs}} \times \frac{1 \text{ cup}}{8 \text{ oz}} = 1 \text{ cup}$$

EXAMPLE   Convert 5 ounces to teaspoons.

           Starting Factor   Answer Unit

               5 oz   tsp

Equivalents: 1 oz = 6 tsp

Conversion Equation:

$$5 \; \cancel{oz} \times \frac{6 \text{ tsp}}{1 \; \cancel{oz}} = 30 \text{ tsp}$$

PRACTICE
Convert within the Household System

1. 1 glass to tsp

2. 2 gal to oz

3. 4 qt to cups

4. 68 in to ft

5. 4 tbs to oz

6. 6 tbs to tsp

7. 22 pts to gal

8. ½ measuring cup to tbs

9. 50 tsp to oz

10. 1 teacup to tbs

(**Note:** See Appendix G for answer key.)

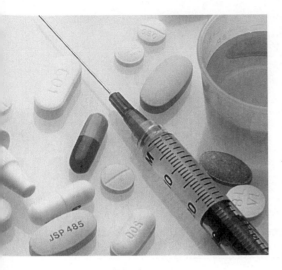

CHAPTER 5

Conversion of Metric, Apothecaries, and Household Units

Upon completion of this chapter you should be able to:

- List approximate equivalent values among the three systems of measurement: metric, apothecaries, and household.
- Apply dimensional analysis to conversions among these systems of measurement.

It is essential that nurses be able to convert accurately among the various systems of measurement, because medication orders often are written in one system and dispensed in another.

Having memorized the basic units and relationships within the metric, apothecaries, and household systems, the learner is now ready to apply dimensional analysis to conversions among these systems. Table 5-1 illustrates the equivalent relationships among the metric, apothecaries, and household systems. Also study Figures 5-1, 5-2, and 5-3 to visualize these relationships.

Self-Quiz—Equivalents

A. Fill in the blanks

1. 60 mg = _____ gr

2. 15 gr = _____ g

3. 1 g = _____ mg

4. 1 kg = _____ g

5. 1 kg = _____ lb

6. 1 ℥ = _____ gtt

7. 1 L = _____ mL

8. 1 in = _____ cm

9. 1 m = _____ in

10. 1 tbs = _____ oz

B. Match equivalent amounts

_____	**1.** 1 mL	**a.**	1 oz
_____	**2.** 1 tsp	**b.**	4 dr
_____	**3.** 1 cup	**c.**	5 mL
_____	**4.** 15 mL	**d.**	15 ɱ
_____	**5.** 30 mL	**e.**	250 mL
		f.	500 mL

(**Note:** See Appendix G for answer key.)

TABLE 5-1   Approximate Equivalents among Metric, Apothecaries, and Household Systems

Metric		Apothecaries		Household
Dry				
60 mg	=	1 gr		
1 g	=	15 gr		
15 g	=	4 dr	=	1 tbs (3 tsp)
30 g	=	1 oz (8 dr)	=	1 oz (2 tbs)
		16 oz	=	1 lb (avoirdupois)
1 kg			=	2.2 lb
Liquid				
1 mL	=	15–16 ɱ	=	15 gtt
4 mL	=	1 dr		
5 mL	=	75 ɱ	=	1 tsp
15 mL	=	4 dr	=	1 tbs (3 tsp)
30 mL	=	1 oz (8 dr)	=	1 oz (2 tbs)
500 mL	=	16 oz (1 pt)	=	16 oz (1 pt or 2 cups)
1000 mL	=	32 oz (1 qt)	=	32 oz (1 qt)
Length				
2.5 cm			=	1 in
1 m			=	39.4 in

FIGURE 5-1   Weight conversions

mg – g – gr

1000 mg = 1 g = 15 gr

60 mg = 1 gr

1000 g = 1 kg = 2.2 lb

FIGURE 5-2 Volume conversions

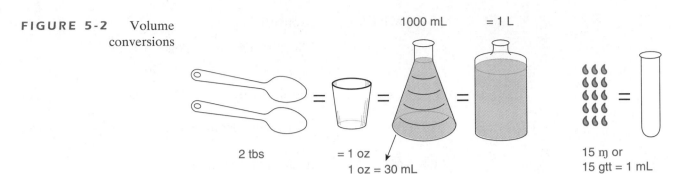

FIGURE 5-3 Length conversions

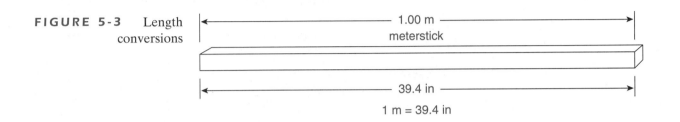

Conversion from One System to Another

EXAMPLE   Convert 5 g to gr

Starting Factor	Answer Unit
5g	gr

Equivalents: 1 g = gr 15

Conversion Equation: $5\,\cancel{g} \times \dfrac{\text{gr }15}{1\,\cancel{g}} = \text{gr }75$

EXAMPLE   Convert 5.4 lb to kg

Starting Factor	Answer Unit
5.4 lb	kg

Equivalents: 1 kg = 2.2 lb

Conversion Equation: $5.4\,\cancel{lb} \times \dfrac{1\text{ kg}}{2.2\,\cancel{lb}} = 2.5\text{ kg}$

EXAMPLE   Convert gr 45 to g

Starting Factor	Answer Unit
gr 45	g

Equivalents: gr 15 = 1 g

Conversion Equation: $\cancel{\text{gr }}45 \times \dfrac{1\text{ g}}{\cancel{\text{gr }}15} = 3\text{ g}$

EXAMPLE   Convert 54 kg to lb

Starting Factor   Answer Unit
54 kg   lb

Equivalents: 2.2 lb = 1 kg

Conversion Equation: $54 \, \cancel{kg} \times \dfrac{2.2 \, lb}{1 \, \cancel{kg}} = 118.8 \, lb$

EXAMPLE   Convert 16 mL to dr

Starting Factor   Answer Unit
16 mL   dr

Equivalents: 4 mL = 1 dr

Conversion Equation: $16 \, \cancel{mL} \times \dfrac{1 \, dr}{4 \, \cancel{mL}} = 4 \, dr$

EXAMPLE   Convert 8 oz to mL

Starting Factor   Answer Unit
8 oz   mL

Equivalents: 1 oz = 30 mL

Conversion Equation: $8 \, \cancel{oz} \times \dfrac{30 \, mL}{1 \, \cancel{oz}} = 240 \, mL$

EXAMPLE   Convert 480 mL to oz

Starting Factor   Answer Unit
480 mL   oz

Equivalents: 30 mL = 1 oz

Conversion Equation: $480 \, \cancel{mL} \times \dfrac{1 \, oz}{30 \, \cancel{mL}} = 16 \, oz$

EXAMPLE   Convert gr 2 ½ to mg

Starting Factor   Answer Unit
gr 2 ½   mg

Equivalents: gr 1 = 60 mg

Conversion Equation: $\cancel{gr} \, 2\frac{1}{2} \times \dfrac{60 \, mg}{\cancel{gr} \, 1} = 150 \, mg$

EXAMPLE   Convert 300 mg to gr

Starting Factor   Answer Unit
300 mg   gr

Equivalents: 60 mg = gr 1

Conversion Equation: $300 \, \cancel{mg} \times \dfrac{gr \, 1}{60 \, \cancel{mg}} = gr \, 5$

EXAMPLE   **j.** Convert 10 mL to tsp

     Starting Factor   Answer Unit

       10 mL   tsp

   Equivalents: 5 mL = 1 tsp

   Conversion Equation: $10 \; \cancel{mL} \times \dfrac{1 \; tsp}{5 \; \cancel{mL}} = 2 \; tsp$

PRACTICE

Carry each answer to two decimal places and round to the nearest tenth

1. 2.5 pts to mL

2. 40 kg to lb

3. 600 mL to cups

4. 2 tsp to mL

5. gr $\overline{ss}$ to mg

6. ℥ 50 to kg

7. ♏ xx to mL

8. ℥ iv to tbs

9. 0.6 L to ℥

10. 2 g to gr

11. ʒ i$\overline{ss}$ to gtt

12. 5 mL to ♏

13. 120 mg to gr

14. 10 gtt to mL

15. 12.5 mL to tsp

16. 1 ½ tbs to mL

17. 2 cups to mL

18. 6 tsp to ʒ

19. 120 gr to g

20. 157 lb to kg

21. gr 3 to mg

22. 3 mL to ♏

23. 5.2 kg to lb

24. 120 mm to cm

25. 60 cm to in

26. 0.5 pt to ʒ

27. 90 mg to gr

28. 5.5 g to gr

29. 60 mL to tbs

30. gr 5 to mg

(**Note:** See Appendix G for answer key.)

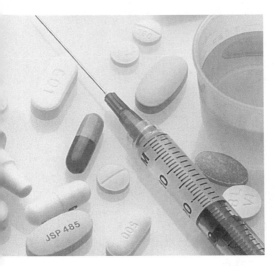

Calculation of Oral Medications

Upon completion of this chapter you should be able to:

- Identify various forms of oral medications.
- Read dosage calibrations on a medicine cup, dropper, and syringe.
- Read drug labels to obtain information about specific drugs administered orally.
- Demonstrate knowledge of the appropriate method of rounding off doses when administering oral medications.
- Apply dimensional analysis to clinical calculations involving oral medications.

Oral Medications

Medications that are administered by mouth and absorbed via the gastrointestinal tract are known as po (per os, by mouth) drugs. It is necessary to become familiar with this abbreviation to administer these drugs by the correct route, which should be designated as po (or o) in the medication order.

A variation of the oral route is called the *sublingual route*, whereby medication is placed under the tongue for absorption via the mucous membrane into the circulatory system. This route is designated by the abbreviation sl in the medication order. When medication is ordered to be administered via the *buccal* route, it is placed between the cheek and gum for similar absorption. Neither sublingual nor buccal medications should be chewed or swallowed whole and, as a rule, are not followed by water.

It is necessary to recognize the various forms in which oral medications are dispensed and to understand how to read labels of medication containers, as well as calibrations on equipment used to dispense liquid medications.

Figure 6-1 illustrates a variety of oral medication forms:

- Tablets—contain a powdered drug compressed into a tablet. Tablets come in various shapes and may be half-scored or quarter-scored. They may be broken or crushed and placed in food for patients who have difficulty swallowing.
- Coated tablets—covered with a flavored coating to facilitate swallowing and disguise taste. They cannot be divided and should not be crushed.
- Enteric coated—covered with a coating that delays dissolution and absorption until tablet reaches the small intestine. They cannot be divided and should not be crushed.

FIGURE 6-1 Oral medication forms

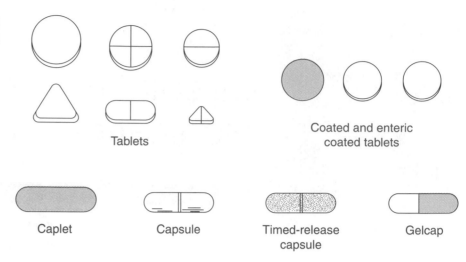

Tablets

Coated and enteric coated tablets

Caplet

Capsule

Timed-release capsule

Gelcap

- Capsules—contain a drug enclosed in a gelatin container to conceal taste. May be opened and contents placed in food, unless this is contraindicated by desired action of the drug.

- Caplet—tablet shaped like a capsule. May be coated. Should not be broken.

- Sustained-release capsules or tablets—drug granules coated to dissolve at different times to provide for continuous release of drug over an extended time period. (Also called timed-release capsules, spansules, tempules, or caplets.) Must never be opened or broken apart before administering.

- Liquids—dispensed as elixirs, syrups, suspensions, or solutions.

The Medicine Cup

The most common type of container used for dispensing fluid drugs is the medicine cup, made of glass or plastic, Figure 6-2. It usually is calibrated in one or more of the three measuring systems: metric, apothecaries, and household.

When a solution is poured into a medicine cup, capillary attraction causes the fluid in contact with the cup to be drawn upward and the surface of the solution becomes concave. The curved surface is called the *meniscus* and the reading of the dose must be made at the lowest point of the meniscus when the cup is held at eye level.

Note that the smallest amounts for which most medicine cups are calibrated are 1 dram, 1 teaspoon, or 5 milliliters. When measuring smaller amounts, it is recommended that the medication be drawn up into a syringe, which facilitates a more accurate measurement. Some liquid medications are premeasured for oral administration in a single-dose syringe.

When pills, tablets, or capsules are being dispensed, they may be placed in a plastic medicine cup or in a small paper (souffle) cup, depending on hospital policy. Many such medications are wrapped individually and should be opened at the bedside just prior to administration.

FIGURE 6-2   Medicine cup

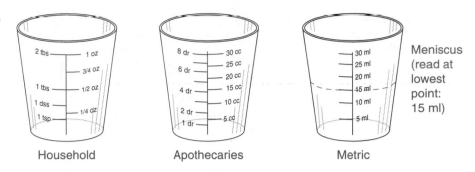

Household   Apothecaries   Metric

Meniscus (read at lowest point: 15 ml)

Rounding Off

When Administering Tablets

- Scored tablets may be broken in half or quarters in order to obtain as exact a dose as possible, Figure 6-1.

  EXAMPLE   If calculated dose is: 1.5 tablets, give 1 ½ tablets

  1.25 tablets, give 1 ¼ tablets

  1.75 tablets, give 1 ¾ tablets

- If tablets are not scored, a pill splitter may be used if hospital policy permits. Because this can be a very inaccurate method, it should be used only when an alternative form (e.g., liquid) of the medication is not available. Check with the pharmacist regarding alternative dosage forms.

- Capsules, spansules, and enteric coated tablets cannot be divided. If the calculated dose is not a whole number, consult with the pharmacist or physician in regard to rounding.

When Administering Liquids

- If measuring in milliliters, carry the calculation to two decimal places and round to the nearest tenth. If the calculated dose is an even multiple of 5, it may be measured in the medicine cup. Any dosage that is not an even multiple of 5 should be measured using a syringe as this permits accurate measurement of small amounts, including tenths of milliliters, Figure 6-3.

  EXAMPLE   If calculated dose is: 2.3 mL, draw up entire amount in syringe

  5 mL, measure in medicine cup

  12.7 mL, pour 10 mL into medicine cup, draw up 2.7 mL into syringe, and add to medication in cup

- If measuring in teaspoons or tablespoons, carry the calculation to two decimal places and round to the nearest tenth. If the calculated dose is

FIGURE 6-3   Measuring liquids

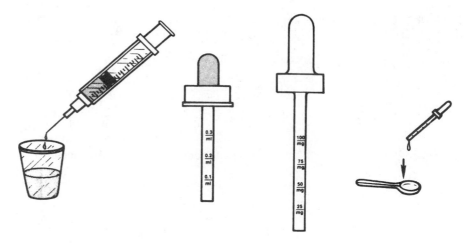

an exact teaspoon or tablespoon, it may be measured in the medicine cup. Any dosage that is not an exact teaspoon or tablespoon should be converted to milliliters and measured as above, using a syringe. This method is more accurate than converting milliliters to drops.

■ Liquid medications often are dispensed with a dropper attached to the bottle cap. This dropper usually is calibrated in milliliters (e.g., 0.1 mL, 0.2 mL) or by actual dosage (e.g., 75 mg, 100 mg), thus facilitating accurate measurement of the medication, Figure 6-3.

■ Medications that are ordered in drops (household system) can be drawn up into a dropper and the required number of drops placed in a spoon or medicine cup for administration, Figure 6-3.

Reading Labels and Calculating Dosage

All medication containers are labeled as to their contents and directions for use. Individuals administering medications must be able to read and understand the information given on the label. This information includes:

■ Name of drug: Trade name—the brand name; the registered trademark assigned by the manufacturer; usually followed by ®. Generic name (by law this must appear on all drug labels)—the official name assigned to a drug; the name under which it is licensed. Drugs that have been in use for many years may thereafter be manufactured and sold under the generic name, eliminating the need for a brand name. Therefore, if only one name appears on a drug label, it is the generic name.

■ Dosage strength: Amount or concentration of the drug—per vial, ampule, mL, tablet, capsule, etc. This may be written in more than one system of measurement (e.g., metric, apothecaries).

■ Name of manufacturer

Some labels may also indicate:

■ Form: Liquid—mL, oz, etc. Solid tablet, capsule, powder, etc.(not always indicated on the label).

- Expiration date: How long the medication (usually liquid) will remain stable or potent.

- Total amount per container: Total volume, if liquid; total number, if solid. It is important not to confuse this number or quantity with the dosage strength of the drug.

- Directions for administering (or storing): mixing, reconstituting, shaking, refrigerating, etc.

Reading Labels

EXAMPLE   Figure 6-4

FIGURE 6-4

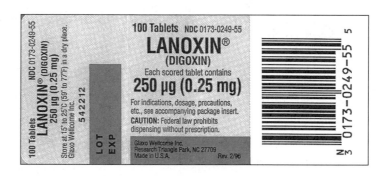

1. Trade Name: Lanoxin

2. Generic Name: Digoxin

3. Dosage Strength: 250 μg, same as 0.25 mg per tablet

4. Form: Tablet

5. Manufacturer's Name: Glaxo Wellcome Inc.

6. Directions for Storage: Store at 15°–25°C, 59°–77°F in a dry place

7. Total Amount per Container: 100 tablets

8. **Order:** Lanoxin 0.5 mg po

   How many tablets should the patient receive?

   Starting Factor   Answer Unit
      0.5 mg   tab

   Equivalent: 0.25 mg = 1 tab

   Conversion Equation: $0.5 \, \text{mg} \times \dfrac{1 \, \text{tab}}{0.25 \, \text{mg}} = 2 \, \text{tab}$

EXAMPLE   Figure 6-5

FIGURE 6-5   *(Courtesy of SmithKline Beecham Pharmaceuticals)*

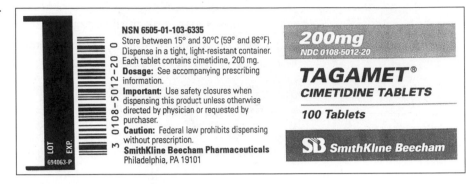

1. Trade Name: Tagamet

2. Generic Name: Cimetidine tablets

3. Dosage Strength: 200 mg tab

4. Form: tablets

5. Manufacturer's Name: SmithKline Beecham

6. **Order:** Tagamet 400 mg po

   How many tablets should the patient receive?

Starting Factor	Answer Unit
400 mg	tab

   Equivalent: 200 mg = 1 tab

   Conversion Equation: $400 \text{ mg} \times \dfrac{1 \text{ tab}}{200 \text{ mg}} = 2 \text{ tab}$

PRACTICE
Reading Labels

A. Figure 6-6

FIGURE 6-6

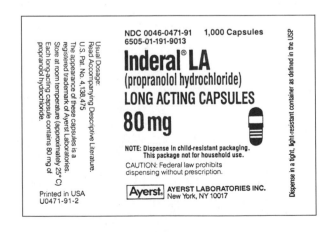

1. Trade Name: _____

2. Generic Name: _____

3. Dosage Strength: _____

4. Form: _____

5. Manufacturer's Name: _____

6. **Order:** Inderal LA 80 mg po

    How many capsules should be administered? _____

7. **Order:** Inderal LA 160 mg po

    How many capsules should be administered? _____

B. Figure 6-7

FIGURE 6-7

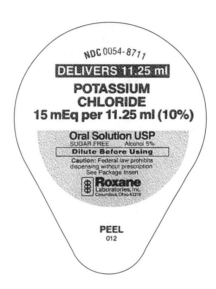

1. Trade Name: _____

2. Generic Name: _____

3. Dosage Strength: _____

4. Form: _____

5. Manufacturer's Name: _____

6. **Order:** KCl 15 mEq po

    How many mL should the patient receive? _____

7. **Order:** KCl 10 mEq po

    How many mL should the patient receive? _____

C. Figure 6-8

FIGURE 6-8

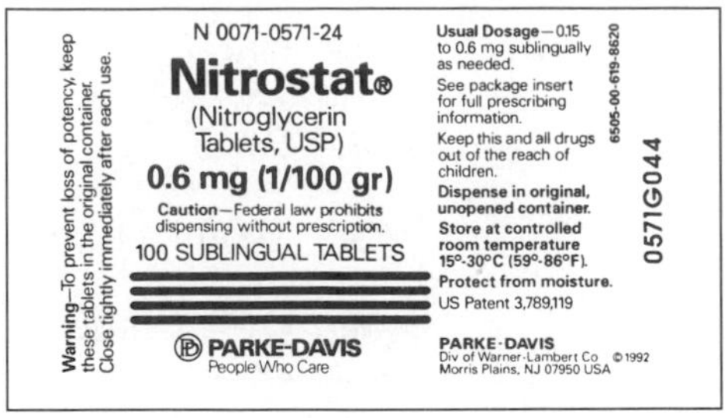

1. Trade Name: _____

2. Generic Name: _____

3. Dosage Strength: _____

4. Form: _____

5. Manufacturer's Name: _____

D. Figure 6-9

FIGURE 6-9

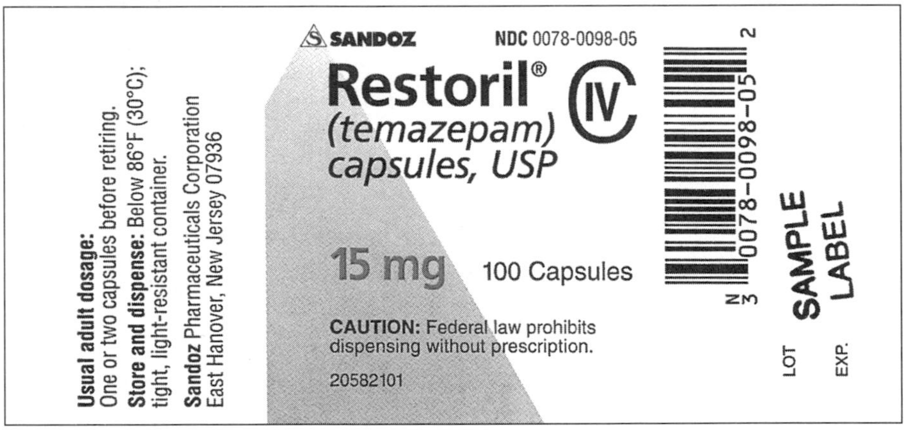

1. Trade Name: _____

2. Generic Name: _____

3. Dosage Strength: _____

4. Form: _____

5. Manufacturer's Name: _____

(**Note:** See Appendix G for answer keys.)

1. **Order:** Prednisone 20 mg po

    Label: Figure 6-10

    How many tablets should be administered? _____

FIGURE 6-10

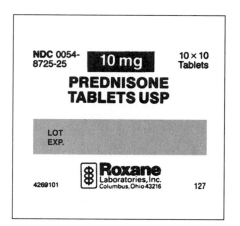

NDC 0054-8725-25   10 mg   10 × 10 Tablets

PREDNISONE TABLETS USP

LOT
EXP.

Roxane Laboratories, Inc. Columbus, Ohio 43216

4269101   127

2. **Order:** Halcion 0.25 mg po

    Label: Figure 6-11

    How many tablets should be administered? _____

FIGURE 6-11

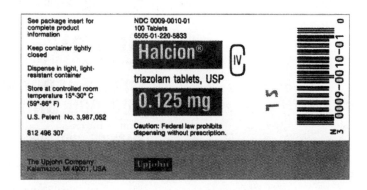

3. **Order:** Hydroxyzine Pamoate 60 mg po

    Label: Figure 6-12

    How many mL should be administered? _____

FIGURE 6-12 *(Courtesy
Pfizer Laboratories Division,
Pfizer Inc.)*

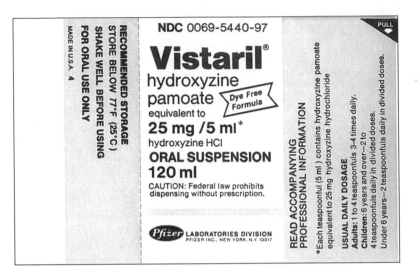

4. **Order:** Nilstat Suspension 1 tsp po

    Label: Figure 6-13. What is the generic name? _____

    How many units should be administered? _____

FIGURE 6-13 *(Courtesy
Lederle Laboratories)*

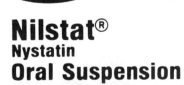

5. **Order:** Compazine 10 mg po

    Label: Figure 6-14. What is the generic name? _____

    How many tablets should be administered? _____

FIGURE 6-14 *(Courtesy of SmithKline Beecham Pharmaceuticals)*

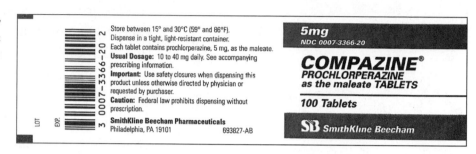

Store between 15° and 30°C (59° and 86°F).
Dispense in a tight, light-resistant container.
Each tablet contains prochlorperazine, 5 mg, as the maleate.
Usual Dosage: 10 to 40 mg daily. See accompanying prescribing information.
Important: Use safety closures when dispensing this product unless otherwise directed by physician or requested by purchaser.
Caution: Federal law prohibits dispensing without prescription.
SmithKline Beecham Pharmaceuticals
Philadelphia, PA 19101   693827-AB

5mg
NDC 0007-3366-20

COMPAZINE®
PROCHLORPERAZINE
as the maleate TABLETS

100 Tablets

SB SmithKline Beecham

(**Note:** See Appendix G for answer key.)

Calculations Based on Body Weight

Medications may be prescribed according to a designated amount of drug per kilogram or pound of body weight. Specific amounts of drug per unit of body weight are recommended by the drug manufacturer, and this information can be found in the product insert or in a drug reference publication. Medication orders may be written in amounts for individual doses or for total daily (24 hr) dosage, in which case the total calculated dosage must be divided by the specified number of doses to be given.

Because the amount of medication to be given is determined by the weight of the person, this weight and the calculated dosage can be considered an equivalent relationship. Our goal is to convert a particular quantity of weight to a corresponding quantity of medication. Therefore, the starting factor is in *lb* or *kg* and the answer label is in whatever units the medication is dispensed (e.g., *mL, mg, tab,* etc.).

EXAMPLE

Order: Thiabendazole Suspension 25 mg/kg/24 hr po to an adult weighing 148 lb

Label: Thiabendazole Suspension 500 mg/5 mL

How many mL should be administered?

    Starting Factor   Answer Unit

       148 lb   mL

Equivalents: 2.2 lb = 1 kg, 25 mg = 1 kg, 500 mg = 5 mL

Conversion Equation:

$$148\ \cancel{lb} \times \frac{1\ \cancel{kg}}{2.2\ \cancel{lb}} \times \frac{25\ \cancel{mg}}{1\ \cancel{kg}} = \frac{5\ mL}{500\ \cancel{mg}} = 16.8\ mL$$

In the first example, the total calculated dosage is administered in one dose. If the order specifies administering the medication in divided doses, it is necessary to divide the total calculated dosage by the number of doses prescribed so that the correct amount per dose will be administered.

EXAMPLE   **Order:** Chloromycetin 50 mg/kg/day in four divided doses po to an adult weighing 80 kg

Label: Chloromycetin (chloramphenicol) 250 mg/cap

How many capsules should be administered *per dose?*

Starting Factor	Answer Unit
80 kg	cap

Equivalents: 50 mg = 1 kg, 1 cap = 250 mg

Conversion Equation:

$$80 \text{ kg} \times \frac{50 \text{ mg}}{1 \text{ kg}} \times \frac{1 \text{ cap}}{250 \text{ mg}} = \frac{16 \text{ cap}}{4 \text{ doses}} = 4 \text{ cap/dose}$$

EXAMPLE   **Order:** Ancobon 50 mg/kg/day in four divided doses po to an adult weighing 135 lb

Label: Ancobon (flucytosine) 250 mg/cap

How many capsules should be administered *per dose?*

Starting Factor	Answer Unit
135 lb	cap

Equivalents: 1 kg = 2.2 lb, 50 mg = 1 kg, 1 cap = 250 mg

Conversion Equation:

$$135 \text{ lb} \times \frac{1 \text{ kg}}{2.2 \text{ lb}} \times \frac{50 \text{ mg}}{1 \text{ kg}} \times \frac{1 \text{ cap}}{250 \text{ mg}} = \frac{12.2 \text{ cap}}{4 \text{ doses}} = 3 \text{ cap/dose}$$

REMEMBER

It is critically important to perform this final step, dividing by number of doses, in computations based on body weight. Consistency in this regard helps avoid errors when medication is to be given in divided doses. If this step is omitted, it is easy to forget to divide the total daily dose into the prescribed number of doses, thus greatly increasing the risk of administering an overdosage.

Although all of the examples in this chapter and Chapters 8 and 10 illustrate calculations of *adult* dosages based on body weight, the same method is used to calculate *pediatric* dosages also based on body weight.

PRACTICE
Oral Dosage Based on Body Weight

1. **Order:** Ethambutol 15 mg/kg/24 hr po to an adult weighing 130 lb
   Label: Ethambutol 400 mg/tab
   How many tablets should be administered per dose? _____

2. **Order:** Flucytosine 50 mg/kg/day po in four divided doses to an adult weighing 69.4 kg
   Label: Flucytosine 250 mg/cap
   How many capsules should be administered per dose? _____

3. **Order:** Antiminth Oral Suspension 11 mg/kg/ po, one dose only, to an adult weighing 146 lb
   Label: Antiminth (pyrantel pamoate) Oral Suspension 50 mg/mL
   How many mL should be administered? _____

4. **Order:** Myambutol 25 mg/kg/24 hr po to an adult weighing 72.7 kg
   Label: Myambutol (ethambutol HCl) 400 mg/tab (scored)
   How many tablets should be administered per dose? _____

5. **Order:** Isoniazid Tablets 5 mg/kg po in two divided doses to an adult weighing 175 lb
   Label: Isoniazid Tablets 100 mg/tab
   How many tablets should be administered per dose? _____

A. Use dimensional analysis and calculate the correct amount to be administered per dose.

1. **Order:** Amoxil Capsule 500 mg po
   Label: Figure 6-15

FIGURE 6-15

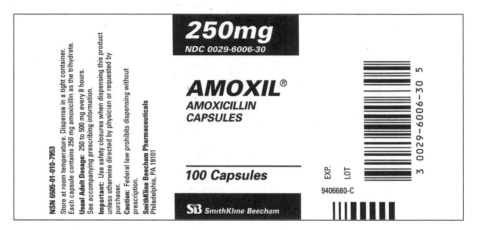

2. **Order:** Xanax 0.5 mg po
   Label: Figure 6-16

FIGURE 6-16

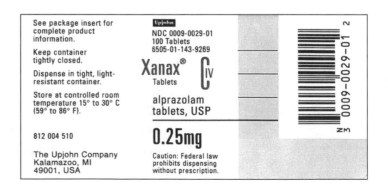

3. **Order:** Ranitidine Hydrochloride 300 mg po
   Label: Figure 6-17

FIGURE 6-17

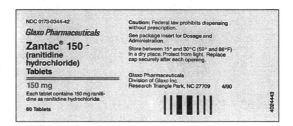

4. Order: Slow-K 32 mEq po
Label: Figure 6-18

FIGURE 6-18

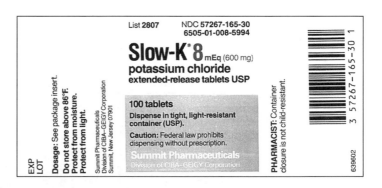

5. Order: Keflex 1 g
Label: Figure 6-19

FIGURE 6-19

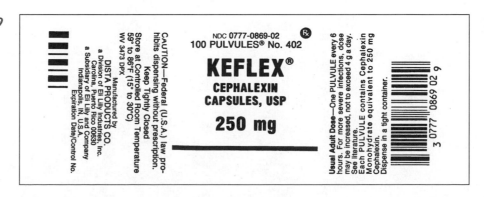

6. **Order:** Digoxin 0.5 mg po
   Label: Figure 6-20

FIGURE 6-20

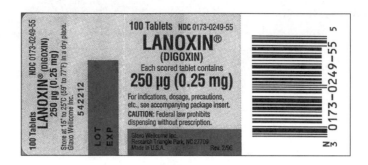

7. **Order:** Ampicillin 0.5 g po
   Label: Figure 6-21

FIGURE 6-21

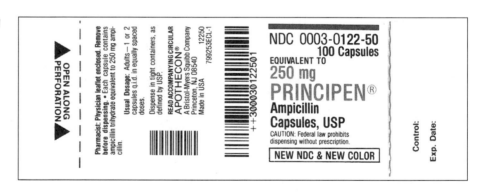

8. **Order:** Meclofenamate Sodium 0.1 g po
   Label: Figure 6-22

FIGURE 6-22

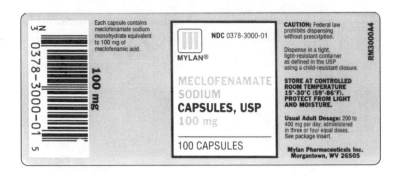

9. **Order:** Penicillin V Potassium Oral Solution 480,000 U po
   Label: Figure 6-23

FIGURE 6-23

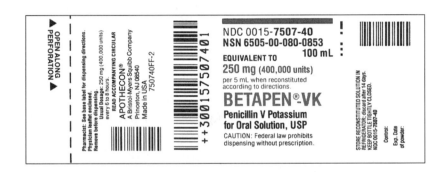

10. **Order:** Danazol Cap 0.4 g po
    Label: Figure 6-24

FIGURE 6-24

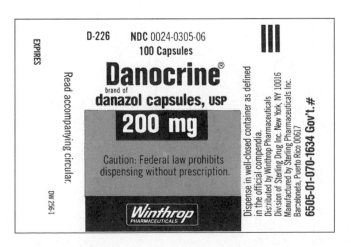

11. The physician ordered Celestone 1.8 mg po. The drug container label states: Celestone (beta-methasone) 0.6 mg/tablet. How many tablets should the patient receive?

12. The physician ordered Erythromycin 150 mg po. The label states: Erythromycin 0.75 g/fluid ounce. How many milliliters should be administered?

13. Aspirin gr 10 po is ordered for the patient. The strength on hand is Aspirin 0.3 g/tablet. How many tablets should be administered?

14. Digoxin Elixir Pediatric 0.12 mg is ordered po. The drug container label states: Digoxin 0.05 mg/mL. How many milliliters should the patient receive?

15. The physician ordered Coumadin gr ⅙ po. How many tablets should the patient receive if the label states: Coumadin (warfarin sodium) 5 mg/tablet?

16. Prolixin 0.125 mg is ordered po. The strength on hand is Prolixin (fluphenazine) 0.25 mg/tablet (scored). How many tablets should be administered?

17. The patient is to receive Penicillin G 400,000 Units po. The drug label states: Penicillin G 800,000 Units/tablet (scored). How many tablets should be administered?

18. The physician ordered Chloral Hydrate gr 15 po hs. The label states: Chloral Hydrate 500 mg/dram. How many ℨ should the patient receive?

19. Nembutal Elixir 60 mg po is ordered. The label states: Nembutal (pentobarbital) Elixir 20 mg/5 mL. How many milliliters should the patient receive?

20. **Order:** Slo-Phylin 75 mg po
    Label: Slo-Phylin (theophylline) 80 mg/15 mL
    How many mL should be administered?

21. **Order:** Aminophylline 300 mg po
    Label: Aminophylline 0.1 g/tab
    How many tablets should the patient receive?

22. **Order:** Azulfidine 1.5 g po
    Label: Azulfidine (sulfasalazine) 500 mg/tab
    How many tablets should be administered?

23. **Order:** Chloromycetin 0.5 g po
    Label: Chloromycetin (chloramphenicol) capsule 250 mg
    How many capsules should the patient receive?

24. **Order:** Feosol Elixir 300 mg po
    Label: Feosol (ferrous sulfate) Elixir 220 mg/5 mL
    How many milliliters should be administered?

25. **Order:** Terramycin 500 mg po
    Label: Terramycin (tetracycline HCl) 50 mg/mL
    How many milliliters should be administered?

26. **Order:** Haldol 1.5 mg po
    Label: Haldol (haloperidol) 0.5 mg/tab
    How many tablets should be administered?

27. **Order:** Sulfisoxazole 0.25 g po
    Label: Sulfisoxazole 500 mg/tab (scored)
    How many tablets should be administered?

28. **Order:** Aldomet 250 mg po
    Label: Aldomet (methyldopa) 1 g/tab (scored in quarters)
    How many tablets should be administered?

29. **Order:** Vibramycin 100 mg po

   Label: Vibramycin (doxycycline) 50 mg/cap

   How many capsules should be administered?

B. Calculate the correct amount per dose.

30. **Order:** KCl 10 mEq po

   Label: Figure 6-25

FIGURE 6-25

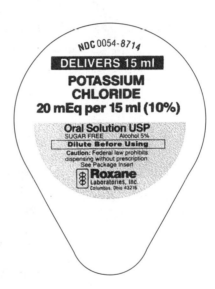

31. **Order:** Cephalexin Capsule 0.5 g po

   Label: Figure 6-26

FIGURE 6-26

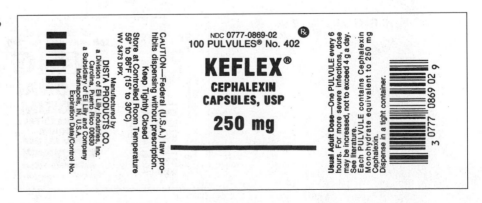

32. **Order:** Codeine Sulfate gr s̄s̄ po
    Label: Figure 6-27

FIGURE 6-27

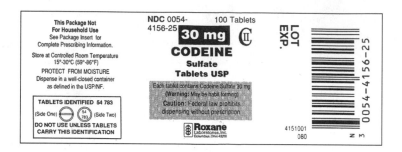

33. **Order:** Phenobarbital gr ¼ po
    Label: Figure 6-28

FIGURE 6-28

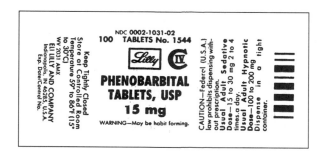

34. **Order:** Seconal Sodium gr īs̄s̄ po
    Label: Figure 6-29

FIGURE 6-29

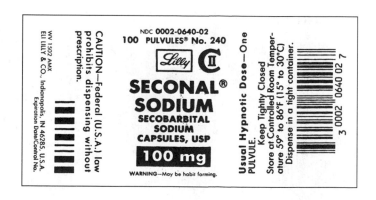

35. **Order:** Tylenol Elixir 60 mg po
    Label: Tylenol (acetaminophen) Elixir 120 mg/5 mL

36. **Order:** Nembutal Sodium gr i$\overline{ss}$ po
    Label: Nembutal Sodium (pentobarbital) 100 mg/cap

37. **Order:** Benadryl Elixir 20 mg po
    Label: Benadryl (diphenhydramine HCl) Elixir 2.5 mg/mL

38. **Order:** Phenergan 0.05 g po
    Label: Phenergan (promethazine HCl) 12.5 mg/tab

39. **Order:** Prolixin 1 mg po
    Label: Prolixin (fluphenazine) 2 mg/tab (scored)

40. **Order:** Gantrisin 750 mg po
    Label: Gantrisin (sulfisoxazole) 0.5 g/tab (scored)

41. **Order:** Compazine Syrup 2.5 mg po
    Label: Compazine (prochlorperazine) Syrup 5 mg/5 mL

42. **Order:** Ascorbic Acid 0.1 g po
    Label: Ascorbic Acid 50 mg/tab

43. **Order:** Dilantin Elixir 100 mg po
    Label: Dilantin (phenytoin sodium) Elixir 125 mg/5 mL

44. **Order:** Dilaudid Cough Syrup 3 mg po
    Label: Dilaudid (dilaudid with guaifenesin) Cough Syrup 1 mg/5 mL
    (Give _____ tsp)

45. **Order:** Mysoline Suspension 125 mg po
    Label: Mysoline (primidone) Suspension 250 mg/5 mL

46. **Order:** Aldomet Oral Suspension 400 mg po
    Label: Aldomet (methyldopa) Oral Suspension 250 mg/5 mL

47. **Order:** Mylicon 80 mg po
    Label: Mylicon (simethicone) 40 mg/0.6 mL

48. **Order:** Mycostatin 1,000,000 U po
    Label: Mycostatin (nystatin) 500,000 U/tab

49. **Order:** Cleocin 150 mg po
    Label: Cleocin (clindamycin) 75 mg/cap

50. **Order:** Synthroid 0.2 mg po
    Label: Synthroid (levothyroxine sodium) 200 mcg/tab

51. **Order:** Mintezol Suspension 25 mg/kg/dose po to an adult weighing 110 lb
    Label: Mintezol (thiabendazole) Suspension 500 mg/5 mL

52. **Order:** Myambutol 25 mg/kg/day to an adult weighing 137 lb
    Label: Myambutol (ethambutol HCl) 400 mg/tab

53. **Order:** Nydrazid 5 mg/kg in two divided doses to an adult weighing 115 lb
    Label: Nydrazid (nystatin) 100 mg/tab

54. **Order:** Trimethoprim 20 mg/kg/24 hr po in four divided doses to an adult weighing 70 kg
    Label: Trimethoprim 160 mg/tab

55. **Order:** Sulfamethoxazole 100 mg/kg/24 hr po in four divided
doses to an adult weighing 154 lb

Label: Sulfamethoxazole 800 mg/tab

How many tablets should be administered per dose?

(**Note:** See Appendix G for answer key.)

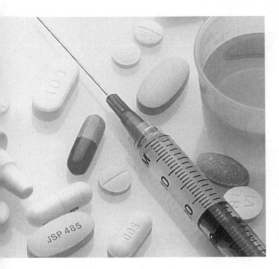

CHAPTER 7

Administration of Oral Medications

OBJECTIVES

Upon completion of this chapter you should be able to:

- Interpret and follow a medication order for the purpose of administering oral medications.
- List the standard abbreviations used in prescribing and administering medications.
- Identify various routes for administering medications.
- List the general rules for safe administration of oral medications: pouring, administering, and recording.
- Identify performance criteria related to administering oral medications.
- Perform a simulated administration of oral medications.

Medication Order
A physician's order is required for medications administered by nurses. This must be a written order signed by the physician. Hospital policies and procedures for medication orders vary, but in most agencies these orders are written on a special form that is a part of the patient's permanent record. The nurse should be sure that a written and signed order exists for any medication given. The only exception to this rule would be under special circumstances, such as emergencies, where a physician may give a verbal order, either directly or by phone. The registered nurse may write the order; the physician must later sign it.

The physician's order (Figure 7-1) consists of the:

1. Patient's name
2. Date and time order is written
3. Name and dosage of medication (**Note:** Name may be written as generic or brand (trade) and dosage may be written in metric, apothecaries, or household systems.)
4. Route of administration
5. Time and frequency of administration
6. Physician's signature

Abbreviations
Many abbreviations are used in prescribing and administering medications. Most of these have been standardized through common usage; however,

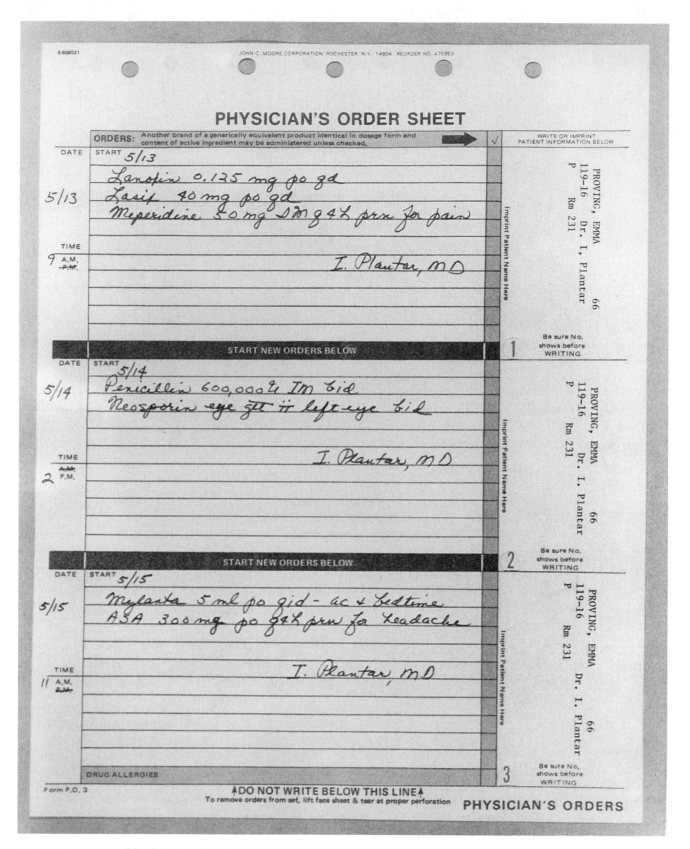

PHYSICIAN'S ORDER SHEET

ORDERS: Another brand of a generically equivalent product identical in dosage form and content of active ingredient may be administered unless checked.

DATE START 5/13

5/13
Lanoxin 0.125 mg po qd
Lasix 40 mg po qd
Meperidine 50 mg IM q4h prn for pain

TIME
9 A.M.
P.M.
I. Plantar, MD

PROVING, EMMA 66
119-16 Dr. I. Plantar
P Rm 231

Be sure No. shows before WRITING

START NEW ORDERS BELOW 1

DATE START 5/14

5/14
Penicillin 600,000 u IM bid
Neosporin eye gtt ii left eye bid

TIME
A.M.
2 P.M.
I. Plantar, MD

PROVING, EMMA 66
119-16 Dr. I. Plantar
P Rm 231

Be sure No. shows before WRITING

START NEW ORDERS BELOW 2

DATE START 5/15

5/15
Mylanta 5 ml po qid - ac + bedtime
ASA 300 mg po q4h prn for headache

TIME
11 A.M.
P.M.
I. Plantar, MD

PROVING, EMMA 66
119-16 Dr. I. Plantar
P Rm 231

Be sure No. shows before WRITING

DRUG ALLERGIES 3

Form P.O. 3

▲DO NOT WRITE BELOW THIS LINE▲
To remove orders from set, lift face sheet & tear at proper perforation

PHYSICIAN'S ORDERS

FIGURE 7-1 Physician's order sheet

occasionally, more than one form is acceptable. To facilitate memorization, commonly used abbreviations have been divided into those dealing with amount or dosage, preparations, routes and times of administration, and any special instructions. Some, which have been introduced in earlier units, are repeated here.

Nurses should know the abbreviations listed in Tables 7-1, 7-2, 7-3, 7-4, and 7-5.

TABLE 7-1   *Amount/Dosage*

Abbreviation	Latin Derivation	English
cc		cubic centimeter
g	gramma	gram
gr	granum	grain
gtt	gutta	drop
lb	libra	pound
ɱ	minimum	minim
mL		milliliter
no	numerus	number
pt	octarius	pint
qs	quantum sifficit	quantity sufficient
ss	semis	one half
ʒ	dracama	dram
ʒ̄	uncia	ounce

TABLE 7-2   *Preparations*

Abbreviation	Latin Derivation	English
cap	capsula	capsule
elix	elixir	elixir
EC		enteric coated
ext	extractum	extract
fl	fluidus	fluid
pil	pilula	pill
sol	solutio	solution
supp	suppositorium	suppository
susp		suspension
syr	syrupus	syrup
tab	tabella	tablet
tr	tincture	tincture
ung	unguentum	ointment

TABLE 7-3   Routes

Abbreviation	Latin Derivation	English
ID		intradermal
IM		intramuscular
IV		intravenous
IVPB		intravenous piggyback
OD	oculus dexter	right eye
OS	oculus sinister	left eye
OU	oculo utro	both eyes
AD	auricula dexter	right ear
AS	auricula sinister	left ear
AU	auriculi utro	both ears
po (o)	per os	by mouth
sc	sub cutis	subcutaneous
sl	sub lingual	sublingual
GT		gastrostomy
NG		nasogastric
NJ		nasojejunal

TABLE 7-4   Times

Abbreviation	Latin Derivation	English
$\overline{a}$	ante	before
ac	ante cibum	before meals
am	ante meridian	before noon
bid	bis in die	*twice a day
h	hora	hour
hs	hora somni	hour of sleep or at bedtime
noct	noctis	night
o	omnis	every
od	omni die	every day
oh	omni hora	every hour
p	post	after
pc	post cibum	after meals
pm	post meridian	after noon
prn	pro re nata	whenever necessary
q	quaque	every
qd	quaque die	every day
qh (q3h, etc.)	quaque hora	*every hour (every 3 hours, etc.)
qid	quater in die	*four times a day
qod		every other day
sos	si opus sit	if necessary (one dose only)
tid	ter in die	three times a day

Note: Medications ordered q2h, q3h, q4h, etc., are given "around the clock" (i.e., throughout a 24-hour period). It is important not to confuse these abbreviations with bid, which means to administer twice a day (not every 2 hours), and qid, which means to administer 4 times a day (not every 4 hours).

TABLE 7-5   Special Instructions

Abbreviation	Latin Derivation	English
aa	ana (Gr.)	of each
ad lib	ad libitum	as desired
c̄	cum	with
dil	dilutus	dilute
per	per	through or by
Rx	recipe	take (or prescription)
s̄	sine	without
stat	statim	immediately

**Self-Quiz—
Abbreviations**

A. Match abbreviations or symbols with correct meaning.

_____ **1.** gtt

_____ **2.** ʒ

_____ **3.** sos

_____ **4.** qh

_____ **5.** ad lib

_____ **6.** bid

_____ **7.** ext

_____ **8.** c̄

_____ **9.** stat

_____ **10.** q

A. as desired

B. dram

C. drop

D. every

E. every hour

F. extract

G. fluid

H. immediately

I. one dose only

J. ounce

K. three times a day

L. twice a day

M. whenever necessary

N. with

B. Write the term.

1. ac   = _____

2. cap   = _____

3. g   = _____

4. pc   = _____

5. q3h   = _____

6. s̄   = _____

7. elix = _____

8. prn   = _____

9. s̄s   = _____

10. mL   = _____

C. Identify the route.

1. IM = _____

2. IV = _____

3. sc = _____

4. OS = _____

5. OD = _____

6. OU = _____

7. po = _____

8. sl = _____

9. ID = _____

(**Note:** See appendix G for answer key.)

Routes for Administering Medications

The common routes by which medications are administered are:

- mouth—po
- swish and swallow—S & S
- gastrointestinal
- injection (parenteral)

    subcutaneous—sc

    intramuscular—IM

    intradermal—ID

    intravenous—IV

    intrathecal (into the spinal canal)

    intracardial (into the heart)   } Less common parenteral

    intra-articular (into a joint)   routes

- inhalation—respiratory tract
- topical—placing on skin, mucous membrane, or in body cavity

    sublingual (under the tongue)

    instillation (dropping liquid into a cavity: eye drops)

    inunction (rubbing ointment on skin)

    irrigation (into a wound or body cavity)

    suppository (vaginal, rectal, urethral)

    patch (applied to the skin, with medication absorbed through the skin)

Medication Administration Record (MAR)

Safe nursing practice requires the use of some type of medication administration record (MAR) or guide to which the nurse can refer when administering medications. Usually this is in the form of a special Kardex, sometimes called a Medex, on which all medication orders for individual patients are reproduced on separate cards or pages. Figure 7-2 is a sample MAR.

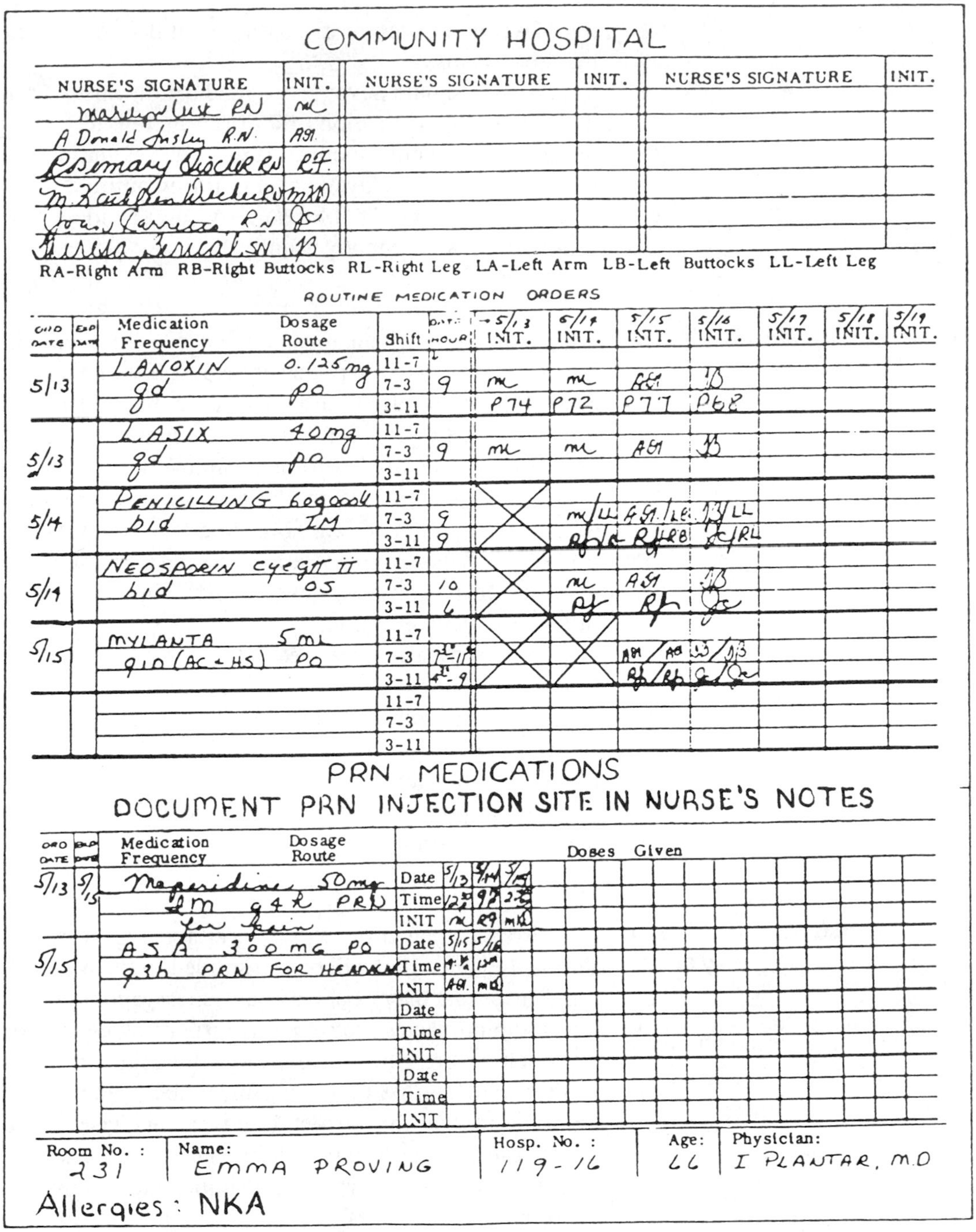

FIGURE 7-2   Medication administration record (MAR)

Note that the patient's name and room number appear on the MAR, along with all pertinent information relating to the order: drug, dose, route, date, and time of administration. As a rule, space for recording each dose given also appears on the record. If pertinent, start and stop dates and special instructions or precautions are included. The presence or absence of allergies should be noted by listing any substance to which the patient is allergic or by using some notation such as NKA (no known allergies). As the MAR is filled up or discontinued, it becomes part of the patient's permanent record.

A nurse should never give a medication without referring to this reproduction of the medication order or, if there is any question, to the original order in the patient's medical record. It is essential that the MAR be up to date and that any delayed or temporarily omitted medication (e.g., patient fasting for test or on call for surgery, etc.) be identified appropriately so it is not administered inadvertently.

Recording Medications

All medications given must be recorded immediately on the patient's MAR, according to the policy of the institution. Only the nurse who administered the medications should sign for them. Usually initials are used for recording, with a place for the full signature somewhere on the sheet or card. Refer to Figure 7-2 for an example of such documentation.

In some institutions, medication order processing and documentation may be computerized; e.g., ordering from pharmacy, billing via business office, recording administration or omission, safety factors such as drug allergies or incompatibilities. Refer to Figure 7-3 for an example of computerized documentation.

There is usually some method for indicating that a medication has been omitted. Whenever this occurs, the reason for the omission should be recorded in the nurse's notes. All narcotics and other controlled drugs must be accounted for on a special record (e.g., narcotic log), again according to the policy of the institution.

The importance of accurate recording of medications cannot be overemphasized.

Drug Distribution System

The physician may order a drug by either its generic name or a brand name. This is the name that will be transcribed to the MAR. Because of the price differences that may exist between generic and brand name products, many hospital pharmacies are currently dispensing generic drugs, insofar as possible. Therefore, the nurse frequently may find a drug labeled by the generic name, rather than the name under which it was ordered. It is essential to verify that the correct drug is being given; a comparison handbook, the *Physician's Desk Reference,* a pharmacist, or some other source should be available for this purpose. The importance of this verification cannot be overemphasized.

The unit dose system is being used more frequently as a method of dispensing drugs. With this method, premeasured drugs are packaged individually and usually are not opened until the time of administration. This method reduces the chance of error, as well as the time spent in preparing and pouring medications. In many instances, the necessity for computation is eliminated, because the drug is dispensed in the same dosage strength as the ordered dose. The nurse still must verify that the correct medication and dose are being administered. Some agencies still may be dispensing medications from labeled containers, rather than unit doses, in which case the nurse has greater responsibility for obtaining and verifying the correct dose.

PATIENT	ACCT #: V008	LOCATION: SNF	UNIT #:	
	AGE/SEX: 84/F	ROOM: 123	REG DATE:	ADM DX:
	STATUS: ADM IN	BED: B	DIS DATE:	

HEIGHT: 4 FT 9 IN 145 CM   WEIGHT: 121 LB OZ 54.88 KG   BSA 1.50   MAR DATE: TO:

ALLERGIES: NO KNOWN DRUG ALLERGIES

MEDICATION		04/29	04/30	05/01	05/02	05/03	05/04	05/05	05/06	05/07	05/08	05/09	05/10	05/11	05/12	05/13
AMLODIPINE BESYLATE 2.5 MG TAB (NORVASC) (None) QD@0730 RX: MC008831 CMTS: 2.5MG PO QD TO CONTROL HYPERTENSION	PO SCH	0730/ ls	/LD	/	/	/	/	/	/	/	/	/	/	/	/	/
POTASSIUM CHLORIDE SOLN 10% 20 MEQ/15 ML (KAOCHLOR SF) (None) 0730 RX: 194819 CMTS: 20MEQ = 15ML POTASSIUM SUPPLEMENT DOSE = 7.5ML (10MEQ) QD IN JUICE	PO SCH	0730/ ls	/LD	/	/	/	/	/	/	/	/	/	/	/	/	/
LANSOPRAZOLE 30 MG CAP (PREVACID) 30 MG (1 CAP) QD@0730 RX: 195816 CMTS: 30 MG PO QD TO CONTROL REFLUX ACID - DO NOT CRUSH IF NECESSARY, CAPSULES MAY BE OPENED AND PUT IN APPLESCAUCE	PO SCH	0730/ ls	/LD	/	/	/	/	/	/	/	/	/	/	/	/	/
TIMOLOL MALEATE OPTH SOLN 0.5% 2.5 ML SO (TIMOPTIC-XE) (None) HS RX: 199959 CMTS: 1 GTT BOTH EYES AT BEDTIME FOR GLAUCOMA. TIMOPTIC XE	OP SCH	2200/ ls	/LD	/	/	/	/	/	/	/	/	/	/	/	/	/

SIGNATURE	INIT.	SIGNATURE	INIT.	SIGNATURE	INIT.	SIGNATURE	INIT.	SIGNATURE	INIT.
Loretta Smith, R.N.	ls								
Joanne Daniels, RN	LD								

FIGURE 7-3   Computerized medication order documentation

Accountability   The nurse is accountable for safe practice in administering medications. This includes questioning and verifying any physician's order that is outside the normal dosage range, as recommended by the drug manufacturer's product insert or a drug reference manual. The nurse should question any medication order that might be contraindicated due to the patient's current condition or that may appear to be having an adverse effect. Moreover, the nurse must be alert for drug allergies, incompatibilities, or interactions, and must have knowledge of appropriate nursing implications and interventions relative to the drugs being administered.

General Rules for Administration of Medications   In the administration of medications, regardless of the route used, the nurse should do the following:

1. Always have a physician's order for medications administered.
2. Wash hands before pouring any medication.
3. Concentrate entirely on preparing and administering medications. Do not allow distractions to interfere with this procedure.
4. Refer to a Medication Administration Record (MAR) for every medication administered, one that corresponds exactly with the physician's order.
5. Check for any known drug allergies the patient might have.
6. If the unit dose system is employed, check the prepackaged unit label against the MAR when obtaining any prepackaged medications from patient's storage area.
7. If a stock or patient supply system is employed, read the label of the medication three times and check with the MAR:
   a. when obtaining the container
   b. just before pouring the medication
   c. immediately after pouring the dose
8. Obtain medications only from legibly labeled containers.
9. Check to be sure the medication is not outdated or has an abnormal appearance.
10. Check the MAR for the time of the most recent administration of a prn medication.
11. Record controlled drugs on the appropriate control sheet when the medication is removed from a locked cupboard.
12. Do not administer medications that have been poured or prepared by another person. **Exception:** If the unit dose system is employed, individual doses will have been dispensed by the pharmacist. The nurse must still verify that the correct medication and dose are administered.
13. Ascertain pertinent information about medications being administered: action, results expected, untoward effects, usual dose, and/or special nursing considerations.
14. Keep the medication cart or tray within sight at all times.

15. Before administering the medication, identify the patient by asking or stating the patient's name, *examining the wristband,* and comparing the information on the wristband to the MAR.

16. If the patient questions or expresses concern about a medication, withhold the medication long enough to recheck the order, the medication, and the dose.

17. If the patient refuses a medication, attempt to ascertain the reason and report and record this information appropriately.

18. Before administering a medication, perform any pertinent assessment relative to the medication; check pulse, blood pressure, respiration, reflexes, pupillary size, etc.

19. Remain with the patient until the medication is taken. Never leave the medication at the patient's bedside without an order from the physician.

20. Maintain an aseptic (clean) technique throughout the procedure.

21. Record the medication immediately after administering it. Observe the patient for desired or undesired effects and report and/or document any pertinent information.

22. Remember the SIX RIGHTS. Administer:
    - the right medication.
    - to the right patient.
    - at the right time.
    - in the right amount.
    - by the right route.
    - with the right documentation.

Administering Oral Medications

In administration of oral medications, it is important to keep in mind the following:

- Check to determine if:

  the dose should be withheld (NPO, nausea, etc.).

  a previously delayed dose that is given once daily may now be administered (test completed, etc.).

  a previously delayed dose that is given several times a day may now be administered according to daily schedule.

- When dispensing prepackaged doses, open the packets at bedside just prior to administration.

- When dispensing pills, tablets, or capsules that are not wrapped, use the cap of the container to transfer the medication into the medicine cup. If possible, the fingers should not come into contact with the drugs.

- If tablets are scored, they may be broken into halves or quarters if necessary. In many agencies, this is done in the pharmacy prior to dispensing.

- If several tablets, pills, or capsules are to be given at one time, they may be poured into the same cup, with the exception of any medications that require assessment prior to administration (e.g., checking pulse, BP, or reflex). These should be poured separately as a reminder or because they may have to be omitted.

- Use a medicine dropper to measure medications ordered in drops.
- In pouring liquid medications, place the thumbnail on the medicine glass marking the correct dose and pour at eye level or with the glass on a flat surface. (Palm label to pour and wipe off lip of bottle, as necessary.)
- The measure of liquid medicine is read at the lowest point of the meniscus.
- Liquid medications may or may not need to be diluted with water or another liquid. Check specific instructions.
- Crush, dissolve, and/or mix medications with small amount of food or liquid as necessary. **Exceptions:** capsules, enteric-coated tablets, or time-release drugs.
- Assist patients to take their medications:

    Elevate head of bed.

    Assess swallowing ability.

    Have water available at bedside.

    If several tablets are to be taken, offer them one at a time.

    Give sips of water after each tablet to increase fluid intake.

    Make sure patient has swallowed all medications.

    Medications administered sublingually, chewables, or medications that should not be followed by water should be given last.

- Record amount of liquid given on Fluid Balance Sheet, if indicated.

The learner may find the following checklist a helpful guide for the administration of oral medications.

Performance Criteria: Administration of Oral Medications

	S	U	Comments
A. Prior to administration 1. Obtains MAR to confirm medication order regarding dose, route, and time of administration			
2. Checks for any known allergies			
3. Washes hands			
B. Administration of tablets or capsules 1. Obtains correct medication			
2. Checks the label against the MAR			
3. a. Pours the correct dose into bottle cap and then into cup; recaps medicine bottle and rechecks label against the MAR			

	S	U	Comments
OR **b.** Selects prepackaged unit dose, checks label against MAR, then places wrapped medication in cup			
4. If controlled drugs are dispensed, maintains security of storage area and documents (records) in appropriate manner			
5. Confirms patient's identity by asking or stating patient's name and checking wristband against MAR			
6. If necessary, assesses pulse, blood pressure, etc. as appropriate for medication being administered			
7. Elevates head, as necessary			
8. Hands the medicine cup to the patient or taps the medicine into the patient's hand or directly into the patient's mouth			
9. Gives water or juice to assist in swallowing medication			
10. For sublingual medication, instructs patient to place tablet under tongue and hold in place until it is absorbed			
11. For buccal medication, instructs patient to place tablet between cheek and teeth, close mouth, and hold tablet against cheek until absorbed			
C. Administration of liquid medications			
1. Obtains correct medication and checks the label against the MAR			
2. Shakes well, if in suspension			
3. Uncaps the bottle and places the cap open side up on a clean surface			

Continues

	S	U	Comments
4. Holds the medicine cup at eye level			
5. Places thumbnail on the correct marking on medicine cup			
6. Pours correct amount of medication, measuring at lowest point of meniscus			
7. Rechecks the poured dosage by setting cup on level surface and reading meniscus at eye level			
8. Rechecks the label against the MAR			
9. Wipes the bottle top with a damp paper towel and replaces cap			
10. Confirms patient's identity by asking or stating name and checking wristband against MAR			
11. Elevates head, as necessary			
12. Hands medicine cup to patient or assists as needed			
a. Uses a straw for medications that stain the teeth (iron, hydrochloric acid, etc.)			
b. Follows medication with water, if indicated			
c. Omits water if contraindicated			
D. Administration of liquid medications via syringe			
1. Obtains correct medication and checks the label against the MAR			
2. Selects correct size syringe according to desired dosage			
3. a. Pours medication into a medicine cup and withdraws the dosage into the syringe **OR**			

	S	U	Comments
b. Withdraws the medication into the syringe via a sterile needle, then discards the needle			
4. Obtains correct dose			
5. Checks dosage in syringe making sure there are no air bubbles displacing medication			
6. Rechecks the label against the MAR			
7. Confirms patient's identity by asking or stating the patient's name and checking wristband against MAR			
8. Places syringe tip inside of patient's mouth and instills the medication slowly			
E. Following administration of medication			
1. Remains with patient until medication is taken			
2. Records accurately on MAR and/or nursing notes			
3. Records fluids given, if indicated			
4. Provides proper after care of equipment			
F. Maintains principles of asepsis throughout the procedure			
G. Maintains principles of patient safety and comfort throughout the procedure			

S—Satisfactory   U—Unsatisfactory   Evaluator _____

The labels in Figure 7-4 represent medications found in a patient's medication storage area. Figure 7-5 is the MAR for this patient.

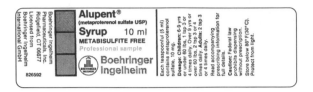

a.

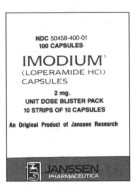

b.

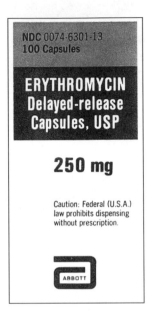

c.

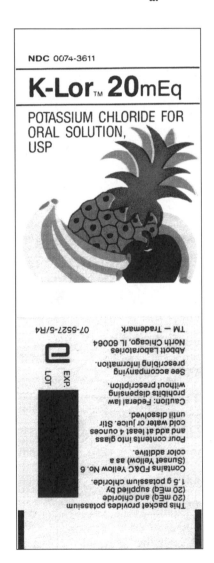

d.

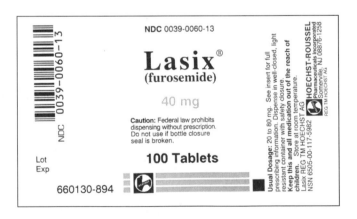

e.

FIGURE 7-4

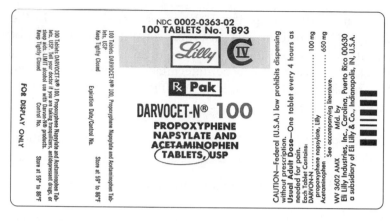

f.

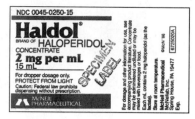

j.

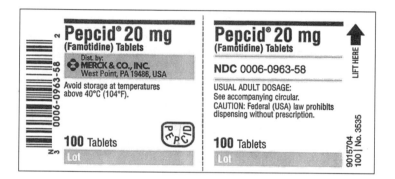

g.

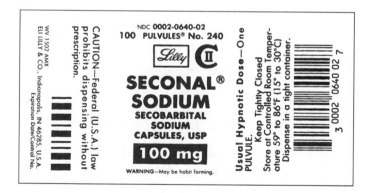

h.

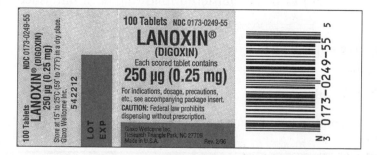

i. Reproduced with permission of Glaxo Wellcome Inc.

FIGURE 7-4   *Continued*

1. Assume you are to administer the 9:00 A.M. oral medications. In the chart on page 83, record the quantity (mL, capsules, tablets, etc.) of each medication you would administer. In some instances no computation is necessary, because it can be determined by inspection of the label or by simple mental arithmetic. When it is necessary to calculate, *use dimensional analysis.*

2. The Lasix is ordered ac breakfast. How many tablets should the patient receive, and when? _____

3. The K-Lor must be dissolved in liquid prior to administration.

   ▪ What liquids can be used? _____

   ▪ How many mL would you record on the fluid intake record? ____

4. What is the dosage strength of the Pepcid? _____

   ▪ How many tablets should be administered at 7:30 A.M.? _____

5. You administered 1.5 tsp of Alupent. Using dimensional analysis, calculate the following:

   ▪ How many mL did the patient receive? _____

   ▪ How many mg did the patient receive? _____

   ▪ The usual adult dose is 20 mg 3–4 times a day. Did this patient receive a safe dose? _____

6. How many mL does the Haldol bottle contain? _____

   ▪ What is the total number of 1.5 mg doses available from this amount? _____

7. What is the dosage strength of the secobarbital capsules? _____

   ▪ How many capsules will the patient receive at bedtime? _____

8. The original medication order for Imodium was written: Give 2 capsules stat and 1 capsule following each unformed stool.

   ▪ How many mg were administered stat? _____

   ▪ How many mg are to be administered following each unformed stool? _____

9. If the patient is complaining of pain, what medication may be administered? _____

   ▪ How often may the patient receive this medication? _____

   ▪ How many tablets would be administered per dose? _____

(**Note:** See Appendix G for answer key.)

COMMUNITY HOSPITAL

NURSE'S SIGNATURE	INIT.	NURSE'S SIGNATURE	INIT.	NURSE'S SIGNATURE	INIT.

RA–Right Arm RB–Right Buttocks RL–Right Leg LA–Left Arm LB–Left Buttocks LL–Left Leg

ROUTINE MEDICATION ORDERS

Ord Date	Exp Date	Medication Frequency	Dosage Route	Shift	Date→ ↓Hour	6/22 Init.	6/23 Init.	6/24 Init.	6/25 Init.	6/26 Init.	6/27 Init.	6/28 Init.
6/22		Digoxin	0.25 mg	11–7								
		qd	po	7–3	9							
				3–11	Pulse							
6/22		Lasix	80 mg	11–7								
		qd	po	7–3	7:30							
				3–11								
6/22		K Lor	20 mEq	11–7								
		tid pc	po	7–3	9-1							
		Dissolve in 4 ℥	water or juice	3–11	6							
6/22		Pepcid	20 mg	11–7								
		bid-ac	po	7–3	7:30							
				3–11	4:30							
6/22		Alupent Syrup	1.5 tsp	11–7								
		qid	po	7–3	9-1							
				3–11	5-9							
6/22		Erythromycin	500 mg	11–7								
		D-R Cap	po	7–3	9							
		bid		3–11	9							
6/22		HALDOL	1.5 mg	11–7								
		tid	po	7–3	9-1							
				3–11	6							
6/22	6/05	Seconal Sodium	100 mg	11–7								
		qd hs	po	7–3								
				3–11	9							

PRN MEDICATION ORDERS

Ord. Date	Exp. Date	Medication Frequency	Dosage Route		Doses Given
6/22		Imodium	ī	Date	
		following each	po	Time	
		unformed stool		INIT	
6/22		Darvocet N-100	ī	Date	
		q 4h prn	po	Time	
		for pain		INIT	

MEDICATION	AMOUNT TO BE GIVEN

FIGURE 7-5 Medication administration record

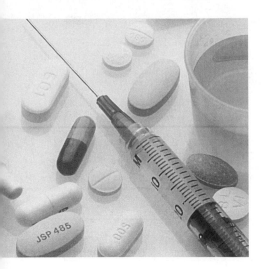

Calculation of Parenteral Medications

Upon completion of this chapter you should be able to:

- Identify appropriate equipment used in the administration of parenteral medications, including types of syringes and the length and gauge of needles.
- Demonstrate the ability to accurately read calibrations on various types of syringes.
- Demonstrate knowledge of the appropriate method for rounding off doses when administering parenteral medications.
- Identify various forms of parenteral medications.
- Read drug labels to obtain information about specific parenteral drugs, including reconstitution.
- Apply dimensional analysis to clinical calculations involving drugs administered by subcutaneous and intramuscular routes.

Parenteral Medications   Medications that are administered via injection into dermal, subcutaneous, or intramuscular tissues or directly into a vein are called parenteral medications, because they are administered by routes outside the gastrointestinal tract.

Parenteral routes include:

1. Intradermal (ID)
2. Subcutaneous (sc)
3. Intramuscular (IM)
4. Intravenous (IV)
5. Intrathecal
6. Intracardial
7. Intra-articular

This chapter focuses on medications administered by intradermal, subcutaneous, and intramuscular routes. Intravenous medications are the subject of Chapters 10 and 11. Intrathecal, intracardial, and intra-articular injections are excluded, because these medication routes require specialized knowledge and training and are beyond the scope of this text.

In this chapter you will learn about the equipment used in administering parenteral medications, the various forms of these medications, and how to read labels and calculate dosages.

The Syringe and Needle

The Syringe

Figure 8-1 illustrates the three parts of a syringe: the barrel holds the medication, is calibrated in tenths (0.1 cc) to measure the quantity to be given, and can range from 0.5 to 50 cc in size. The plunger is made of clouded or colored glass or plastic and is operated to fill or empty the barrel. The lower end of the syringe terminates in a hub to which the needle is attached. It is essential that all parts of the syringe that contact the medication be kept free of contamination. This includes the needle, the outer edge of the hub, the plunger, and the inside of the barrel.

There are various types of syringes available, most of which, at present, are single-use disposable units with attached needles. The needle usually can be detached and replaced. These syringes are made of plastic and are prepackaged in sterile packets. Reusable glass syringes are available, but their use is limited due to the increasing utilization of disposable equipment.

The syringe of choice depends on the route, action, and volume of medication to be administered.

The Tuberculin Syringe The tuberculin syringe measures a total of 1 cc, and is calibrated in hundredths (0.01 cc) and also in minims (16 ɱ/cc). This syringe is used when very small quantities of medication must be measured (i.e., less than 1 cc). It usually is prepackaged with a ⅝″ long needle, Figure 8-2.

The Insulin Syringe The insulin syringe is calibrated in units and should be used exclusively in the administration of insulin, because it will give the most accurate measurement (see Figure 8-3).

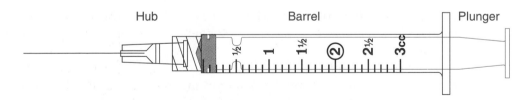

FIGURE 8-1   3 cc syringe

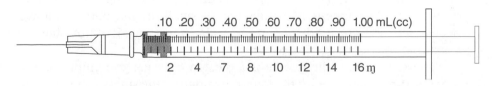

FIGURE 8-2   Tuberculin syringe

FIGURE 8-3   Insulin
syringe

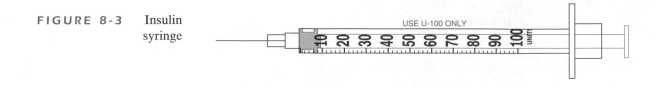

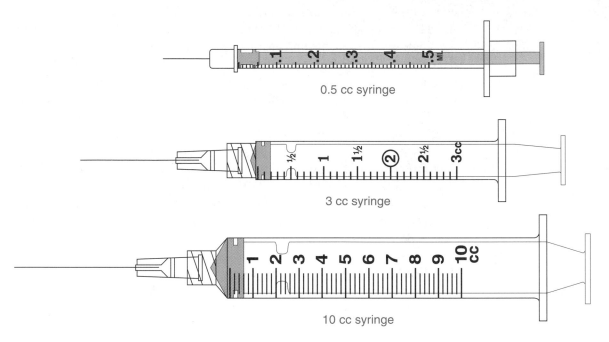

0.5 cc syringe

3 cc syringe

10 cc syringe

FIGURE 8-4   Syringe calibrations

The 0.5, 3, and 10 cc Syringes   The 0.5 cc and 3 cc syringes are calibrated in tenths (0.1 cc) and also in minims. Note that on the cc side, each calibration line measures 0.1 cc.

Ten cc syringes may be used when a large volume of medication is to be measured or administered. It is important to note that on the 10 cc syringe each calibration line measures 0.2 cc, Figure 8-4.

The Needle

The choice of needle depends on the route and site of administration, the size and obesity of the patient, and the viscosity of the medication. Needles vary in length from ¼″ to 3″. Shorter needles (¼″–1″) are used for intradermal or subcutaneous injections and/or small or thin patients; longer needles (1″–2″) are used for intramuscular injections, irritating medications, and/or larger or obese patients.

The diameter of the needle is indicated by a gauge number. Gauge number runs from 14 to 27; the larger the number the smaller the diameter of the needle. Fine needles are used for aqueous solutions and heavier nee-

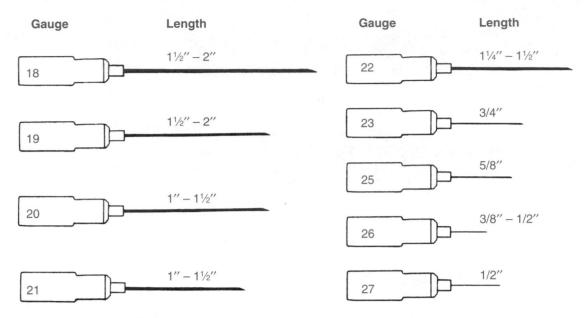

Gauge		Length		Gauge		Length

18 1½″ – 2″

19 1½″ – 2″

20 1″ – 1½″

21 1″ – 1½″

22 1¼″ – 1½″

23 3/4″

25 5/8″

26 3/8″ – 1/2″

27 1/2″

FIGURE 8-5 Needles

dles for suspensions and oils. The widened portion of the needle, called the hub, attaches to the syringe. The angled point, which is called the bevel, increases the sharpness of the needle. A protective cap is provided to maintain sterility. Most needles are now disposable and are destroyed after a single use, Figure 8-5.

Reading the Syringe On most single-use syringes the plunger has a rubber tip that has two rings in contact with the barrel, Figure 8-6. Measurement must be made at the top ring—the one closest to the tip—in order to have an accurate dose. Refer to Figure 8-7.

1. The 3 cc syringe contains 1.2 mL of solution.
2. The tuberculin syringe contains 0.74 mL of solution.
3. The insulin syringe contains 30 units of solution.

FIGURE 8-6 Reading the syringe

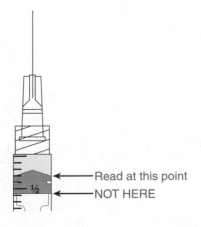

Read at this point

NOT HERE

No. 1

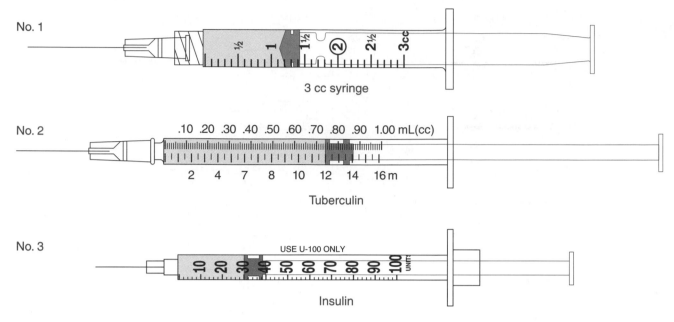

3 cc syringe

No. 2

.10 .20 .30 .40 .50 .60 .70 .80 .90 1.00 mL(cc)

2   4   7   8   10   12   14   16 m

Tuberculin

No. 3

USE U-100 ONLY

10 20 30 40 50 60 70 80 90 100 UNITS

Insulin

FIGURE 8-7 Reading of 3 syringes

Shade in the dosage on the following syringes: Refer to Figure 8-8.

1. 0.6 mL
2. 0.52 mL
3. 64 units

(**Note:** See Appendix G for answer key.)

No. 1

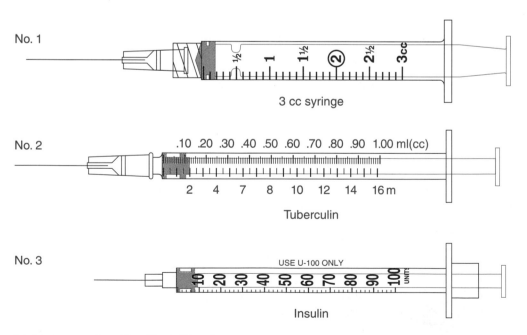

3 cc syringe

No. 2

.10 .20 .30 .40 .50 .60 .70 .80 .90 1.00 ml(cc)

2   4   7   8   10   12   14   16 m

Tuberculin

No. 3

USE U-100 ONLY

10 20 30 40 50 60 70 80 90 100 UNITS

Insulin

FIGURE 8-8 Reading of 3 syringes

Rounding Off Because clinical calculations do not always result in dosages of whole numbers, it is necessary to use the correct procedure for rounding off these values.

- When the calculated dose is obtained in exact tenths of milliliters, the solution may be accurately measured in a 0.5 or 3 milliliter syringe calibrated in tenths; refer to Figure 8-9.

    1. 0.8 mL

    2. 1.3 mL

    3. 2.2 mL

- When the calculated dosage does not result in exact tenths of milliliters, the decimal result is carried to hundredths and rounded in the following manner:

    If the digit in the hundredths place is less than 5, this digit is dropped.

    If the digit in the hundredths place is 5 or greater, the tenths digit is increased by 1.

    These dosages can be administered in a syringe of suitable capacity, calibrated in tenths of milliliters. For example:

    1. 2.31 mL; give 2.3 mL

    2. 1.87 mL; give 1.9 mL

    3. 1.25 mL; give 1.3 mL

    If a tuberculin syringe is used, it is possible to measure hundredths of a milliliter. Therefore, the computation should be carried to thousandths and then rounded to hundredths.

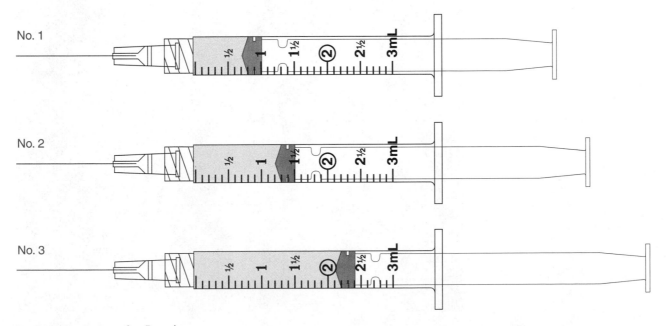

FIGURE 8-9   3 mL syringe

Parenteral Medication Forms

Drugs for parenteral administration are available in a variety of forms. Some come in powder form and must be reconstituted to a liquid, whereas others are in solution and are dispensed in ampules, vials, or cartridges.

Single-Dose Ampules

Most ampules have a constricted stem that facilitates snapping them open. For protection, a piece of gauze or alcohol wipe may be wrapped around the stem before it is broken (Figure 8-10). Any medication in the stem should be shaken down into the ampule before opening. A metal file or an ampule opener can be used to ensure an even break if the ampule is not prescored.

Single- and Multiple-Dose Vials

Some drugs are dispensed in single-dose vials, whereas others are in vials containing several doses. The vial is entered through the rubber diaphragm, which should be cleansed first with an antiseptic. An amount of air comparable to the amount of drug to be withdrawn is injected. The solution can then be withdrawn easily, because fluids move from an area of greater pressure to that of a lesser pressure. It is essential that there be no air bubbles present in the measured quantity, in order to have an accurate dose (Figure 8-11).

Prefilled Cartridges

Some medications are dispensed in premeasured, single-dose disposable cartridges. There may or may not be a needle attached to the cartridge. The prefilled unit is advantageous as a time-saver and reduced risk of contami-

FIGURE 8-10A,B
Obtaining medication from an ampule

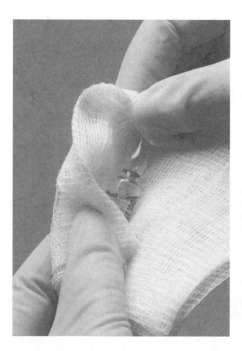
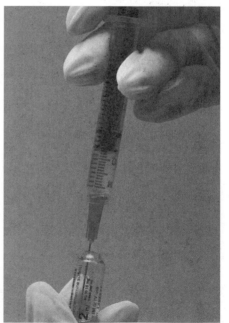

a.   b.

FIGURE 8-11 Obtaining medication from a vial

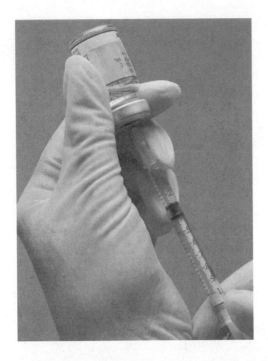

FIGURE 8-12 Pre-filled closed injection systems

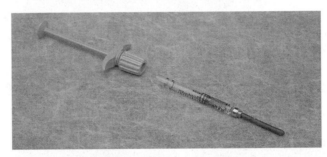

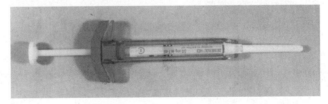

nation. The unit is placed into a cartridge holder or injector, which functions like a syringe. Excess air must be expelled from the cartridge prior to administering the medication. The cartridge holder is reusable; the cartridge and needles are discarded after the medication is administered.

To lessen the risk of needle-stick injuries, the newer injectors are designed to eliminate the need for handling or manipulating the used cartridge or needle, Figure 8-12.

Reading Labels The manufacturer's product insert describes, in detail, the composition of the drug, its actions, indications and contraindications for use, precautions and adverse reactions, dosage, directions for dilution or reconstitution, if necessary, and directions for administration. Figure 8-13 contains excerpts from a manufacturer's product insert.

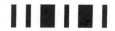

TICAR®
brand of
sterile ticarcillin disodium
for Intramuscular or Intravenous Administration

TR:L4IV

PRESCRIBING
INFORMATION

9608600

DESCRIPTION

Ticar is a semisynthetic injectable penicillin derived from the penicillin nucleus, 6-aminopenicillanic acid. Chemically, it is *N*-(2-Carboxy-3,3-dimethyl-7-oxo-4-thia-1-azabicyclo[3.2.0]hept-6-yl)-3-thiophenemalonamic acid disodium salt.

It is supplied as a white to pale yellow powder for reconstitution. The reconstituted solution is clear, colorless or pale yellow, having a pH of 6.0 to 8.0. Ticarcillin is very soluble in water; its solubility is greater than 600 mg/mL.

ACTIONS

Pharmacology

Ticarcillin is not absorbed orally; therefore, it must be given intravenously or intramuscularly. Following intramuscular administration, peak serum concentrations occur within 1/2 to 1 hour. Somewhat higher and more prolonged serum levels can be achieved with the concurrent administration of probenecid.

The minimum inhibitory concentrations (MICs) for many strains of *Pseudomonas* are relatively high by usual standards; serum levels of 60 mcg/mL or greater are required. However, the low degree of toxicity of ticarcillin permits the use of doses large enough to achieve inhibitory levels for these strains in serum or tissues. Other susceptible organisms usually require serum levels in the 10 to 25 mcg/mL range.

• • •

INDICATIONS

Ticar is indicated for the treatment of the following infections:
   Bacterial septicemia‡
   Skin and soft-tissue infections‡
   Acute and chronic respiratory tract infections‡§
   ‡Caused by susceptible strains of *Pseudomonas aeruginosa, Proteus* species (both indole-positive and indole-negative) and *Escherichia coli.*
   §Though clinical improvement has been shown, bacteriological cures cannot be expected in patients with chronic respiratory disease or cystic fibrosis.
   Genitourinary tract infections (complicated and uncomplicated) due to susceptible strains of *Pseudomonas aeruginosa, Proteus* species (both indole-positive and indole-negative), *Escherichia coli, Enterobacter* and *Streptococcus faecalis* (enterococcus).
Ticarcillin is also indicated in the treatment of the following infections due to susceptible anaerobic bacteria:
1. Bacterial septicemia.
2. Lower respiratory tract infections such as empyema, anaerobic pneumonitis and lung abscess.
3. Intra-abdominal infections such as peritonitis and intra-abdominal abscess (typically resulting from anaerobic organisms resident in the normal gastrointestinal tract).
4. Infections of the female pelvis and genital tract, such as endometritis, pelvic inflammatory disease, pelvic abscess and salpingitis.
5. Skin and soft-tissue infections.
Although ticarcillin is primarily indicated in gram-negative infections, its *in vitro* activity against gram-positive organisms should be considered in treating infections caused by both gram-negative and gram-positive organisms (see Microbiology).
Based on the *in vitro* synergism between ticarcillin and gentamicin sulfate, tobramycin sulfate or amikacin sulfate against certain strains of *Pseudomonas aeruginosa,* combined therapy has been successful, using full therapeutic dosages. (For additional prescribing information, see the gentamicin sulfate, tobramycin sulfate and amikacin sulfate package inserts.)
NOTE: Culturing and susceptibility testing should be performed initially and during treatment to monitor the effectiveness of therapy and the susceptibility of the bacteria.

CONTRAINDICATIONS

A history of allergic reaction to any of the penicillins is a contraindication.

WARNINGS

Serious and occasionally fatal hypersensitivity (anaphylactoid) reactions have been reported in patients receiving penicillin. These reactions are more likely to occur in persons with a history of sensitivity to multiple allergens.
There are reports of patients with a history of penicillin hypersensitivity reactions who experience severe hypersensitivity reactions when treated with a cephalosporin. Before therapy with a penicillin, careful inquiry should be made about previous hypersensitivity reactions to penicillins, cephalosporins and other allergens. If a reaction occurs, the drug should be discontinued unless, in the opinion of the physician, the condition being treated is life-threatening and amenable only to ticarcillin therapy. **Serious anaphylactoid reactions require immediate emergency treatment with epinephrine. Oxygen, intravenous steroids and airway management, including intubation, should also be administered as indicated.**

• • •

FIGURE 8-13   Manufacturer's product insert *(Courtesy of SmithKline Beecham Pharmaceuticals)*

PRECAUTIONS

Although *Ticar* exhibits the characteristic low toxicity of the penicillins, as with any other potent agent, it is advisable to check periodically for organ system dysfunction (including renal, hepatic and hematopoietic) during prolonged treatment. If overgrowth of resistant organisms occurs, the appropriate therapy should be initiated.

Since the theoretical sodium content is 5.2 mEq (120 mg) per gram of ticarcillin, and the actual vial content can be as high as 6.5 mEq/gram, electrolyte and cardiac status should be monitored carefully.

In a few patients receiving intravenous ticarcillin, hypokalemia has been reported. Serum potassium should be measured periodically, and, if necessary, corrective therapy should be implemented.

As with any penicillin, the possibility of an allergic response, including anaphylaxis, exists, particularly in hypersensitive patients.

Usage During Pregnancy

Reproduction studies have been performed in mice and rats and have revealed no evidence of impaired fertility or harm to the fetus due to ticarcillin. There are no well-controlled studies in pregnant women, but investigational experience does not include any positive evidence of adverse effects on the fetus. Although there is no clearly defined risk, such experience cannot exclude the possibility of infrequent or subtle damage to the fetus. Ticarcillin should be used in pregnant women only when clearly needed.

ADVERSE REACTIONS

The following adverse reactions may occur:

Hypersensitivity Reactions: Skin rashes, pruritus, urticaria, drug fever.

Gastrointestinal Disturbances: Nausea and vomiting, pseudomembranous colitis. Onset of pseudomembranous colitis symptoms may occur during or after antibiotic treatment. (See WARNINGS.)

Hemic and Lymphatic Systems: As with other penicillins, anemia, thrombocytopenia, leukopenia, neutropenia and eosinophilia.

Abnormalities of Blood, Hepatic and Renal Laboratory Studies: As with other semisynthetic penicillins, SGOT and SGPT elevations have been reported. To date, clinical manifestations of hepatic or renal disorders have not been observed which could be ascribed solely to ticarcillin.

CNS: Patients, especially those with impaired renal function, may experience convulsions or neuromuscular excitability when very high doses of the drug are administered.

Other: Local reactions such as pain (rarely accompanied by induration) at the site of the injection have been reported. Vein irritation and phlebitis can occur, particularly when undiluted solution is directly injected into the vein.

DOSAGE AND ADMINISTRATION

Clinical experience indicates that in serious urinary tract and systemic infections, intravenous therapy in the higher doses should be used. Intramuscular injections should not exceed 2 grams per injection.

Adults:

Bacterial septicemia	200 to 300 mg/kg/day by I.V. infusion in divided doses every 4 or 6 hours.
Respiratory tract infections	(The usual dose is 3 grams given every 4 hours [18 grams/day] or 4 grams given every 6 hours
Skin and soft-tissue infections	[16 grams/day] depending on weight and the severity of the infection.)
Intra-abdominal infections	
Infections of the female pelvis and genital tract	
Urinary tract infections	
Complicated:	150 to 200 mg/kg/day by I.V. infusion in divided doses every 4 or 6 hours.
	(Usual recommended dosage for average [70 kg] adults: 3 grams q.i.d.)
Uncomplicated:	1 gram I.M. or direct I.V. every 6 hours.

• • •

Children under 40 kg (88 lbs):

The daily dose for children should not exceed the adult dosage.	
Bacterial septicemia	200 to 300 mg/kg/day by I.V. infusion in divided doses every 4 or 6 hours.
Respiratory tract infections	
Skin and soft-tissue infections	
Intra-abdominal infections	
Infections of the female pelvis and genital tract	
Urinary tract infections	
Complicated:	150 to 200 mg/kg/day by I.V. infusion in divided doses every 4 or 6 hours.
Uncomplicated:	50 to 100 mg/kg/day I.M. or direct I.V. in divided doses every 6 or 8 hours.

• • •

DIRECTIONS FOR USE
1 gram, 3 gram and 6 gram Standard Vials

Intramuscular Use (concentration of approximately 385 mg/mL): For initial reconstitution use Sterile Water for Injection, USP, Sodium Chloride Injection, USP, or 1% Lidocaine Hydrochloride solution‡ (without epinephrine):

Each gram of ticarcillin should be reconstituted with 2 mL of Sterile Water for Injection, USP, Sodium Chloride Injection, USP, or 1% Lidocaine Hydrochloride solution‡ (without epinephrine) and **used promptly.** Each 2.6 mL of the resulting solution will then contain 1 gram of ticarcillin.

‡For full product information, refer to manufacturer's package insert for Lidocaine Hydrochloride.

Only the 1 gram vial should be used for intramuscular administration. As with all intramuscular preparations, Ticar (ticarcillin disodium) should be injected well within the body of a relatively large muscle using usual techniques and precautions.

Intravenous Administration (concentration of approximately 200 mg/mL): For initial reconstitution use Sodium Chloride Injection, USP, Dextrose Injection 5% or Lactated Ringer's Injection.

Reconstitute each gram of ticarcillin with 4 mL of the appropriate diluent. After the addition of 4 mL of diluent per gram of ticarcillin, each 1.0 mL of the resulting solution will have an approximate concentration of 200 mg. Once dissolved, further dilute if desired.

Direct Intravenous Injection: In order to avoid vein irritation, administer solution as slowly as possible.

Intravenous Infusion: Administer by continuous or intermittent intravenous drip. Intermittent infusion should be administered over a 30 minute to 2-hour period in equally divided doses.

3 gram Piggyback Bottle

Intravenous Infusion (concentrations of approximately 29 mg/mL to 100 mg/mL): The 3 gram bottle should be reconstituted with a minimum of 30 mL of the desired intravenous solution listed below.

Amount of Diluent	Concentration of Solution
100 mL	1 gram/34 mL (~29 mg/mL)
60 mL	1 gram/20 mL (50 mg/mL)
30 mL	1 gram/10 mL (100 mg/mL)

In order to avoid vein irritation, the solution should be administered as slowly as possible. A dilution of approximately 50 mg/mL or more will further reduce the incidence of vein irritation.

Intravenous Infusion: Stability studies in the intravenous solutions listed below indicate that ticarcillin disodium will provide sufficient activity between 21° and 24°C (70° and 75°F) within the stated time periods at concentrations between 10 mg/mL and 50 mg/mL — see Stability Period section below.

After reconstitution and prior to administration *Ticar* as with other parenteral drugs should be inspected visually for particulate matter and discoloration.

• • •

©SmithKline Beecham, 1994
SmithKline Beecham Pharmaceuticals
Philadelphia, PA 19101
TR:L4IV
9608600

Printed in U.S.A.

FIGURE 8-13 *(Continued)*

PRACTICE
Reading Labels

FIGURE 8-14

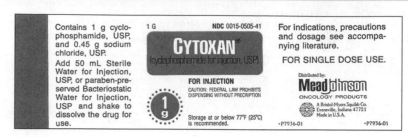

1. Figure 8-14—Circle the generic name and answer the following questions.

    a. What is the total amount of drug in the container? _____

    b. How many mL of diluting solution should be added to the vial for injection? _____

    c. What is the dosage strength of the prepared solution? _____

FIGURE 8-15

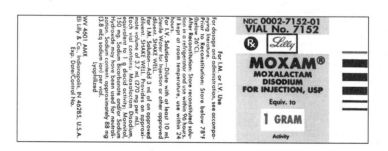

2. Figure 8-15—Circle the trade name and answer the following questions.

    a. By what route(s) can this medication be given? _____

    b. How many mL of diluting solution should be added for IV administration? _____

    c. After the diluent is added to the vial, what is the IM dosage strength of the resulting solution? _____

FIGURE 8-16

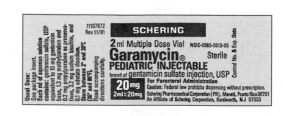

3. Figure 8-16—Circle the total amount of drug in the vial and answer the following questions.

    a. What is the dosage strength of the solution? _____

    b. What is the generic name? _____

    c. Who is the manufacturer? _____

FIGURE 8-17

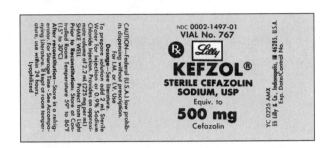

4. Figure 8-17—Circle the generic name and answer the following questions.

    a. How many mL of diluting solution should be added to the vial? _____

    b. What is the dosage strength of the prepared solution? _____

    c. After reconstitution, where should the solution be stored? _____

FIGURE 8-18

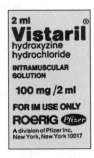

5. Figure 8-18—Circle the route of administration and answer the following questions.

    a. How many mg of medication are contained in 2 mL? _____

    b. By what route only can this medication be given? _____

    c. What is the trade name of this drug? _____

FIGURE 8-19

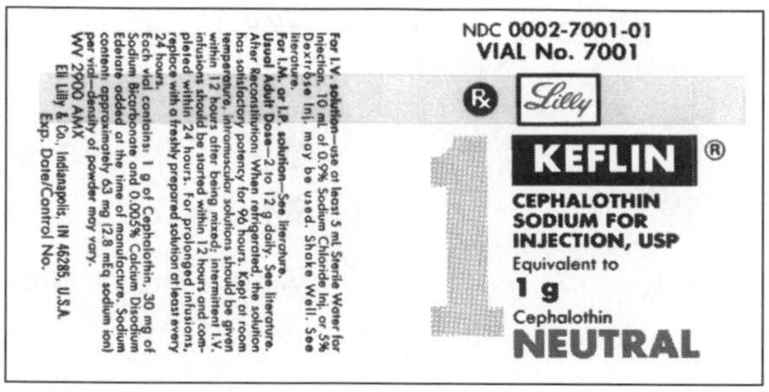

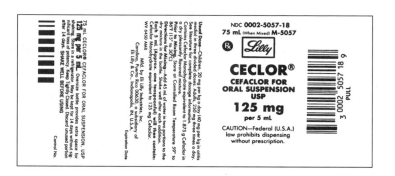

6. Figure 8-19—Circle the usual adult dose and answer the following questions.

    a. How much sterile water should be added to administer this medication IV? _____

    b. What other two solutions can be used to prepare this medication for IV use? _____

    c. By which route(s) can this medication be given? _____

FIGURE 8-20

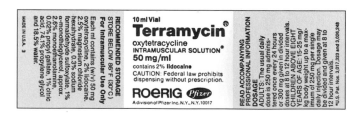

7. Figure 8-20—Circle the trade name and answer the following questions. (Note: This is an oral medication.)

    a. Is this a single or multiple dose container? _____

    b. What is the usual dose for children? _____

    c. What is the dosage strength of this medication? _____

FIGURE 8-21

8. Figure 8-21—Circle the total amount contained in the vial and answer the following questions.

    a. What is the dosage strength of this medication? _____

    b. What is the generic name? _____

    c. Who manufactures this product? _____

FIGURE 8-22

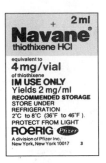

9. Figure 8-22—Circle the generic name and answer the following questions.

   a. By what route *only* can the medication be given? _____

   b. Can the reconstituted solution be stored at room temperature? _____

   c. What is the total amount (volume) of solution in the vial? _____

(**Note:** See Appendix G for answer key.)

Calculating Dosages Obtained from Premixed Solutions

Many parenteral drugs are dispensed in vials or ampules that contain single or multiple doses. The label or printing on each container indicates the amount and the solution strength of the contents. Using these values as equivalents, dimensional analysis can be used to calculate the quantity of solution needed for the required dosage.

FIGURE 8-23

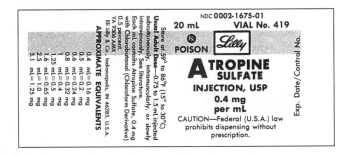

EXAMPLE

A prescription order states: Atropine Sulfate gr $\frac{1}{150}$ IM. The vial of atropine (Figure 8-23) is labeled: Atropine Sulfate 0.4 mg per mL. How much solution will be administered?

Equivalents: gr 1 = 60 mg, 1 mL = 0.4 mg

Conversion Equation:

$$\text{gr } 1/150 \times \frac{60 \text{ mg}}{\text{gr } 1} \times \frac{1 \text{ mL}}{0.4 \text{ mg}} = 1 \text{ mL}$$

OR

$$\text{gr } 0.007 \times \frac{60 \text{ mg}}{\text{gr } 1} \times \frac{1 \text{ mL}}{0.4 \text{ mg}} = 1.05 = 1.1 \text{ mL}$$

FIGURE 8-24

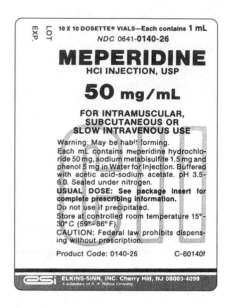

EXAMPLE

The physician orders Demerol 20 mg IM. The medication is dispensed under the label Meperidine 50 mg/mL (Figure 8-24). Find the quantity of solution to be administered.

1. First: Consult a drug reference source to determine that Demerol is a brand name for the generic drug meperidine.

2. Equivalents: 1 mL = 50 mg

Conversion Equation: $20 \text{ mg} \times \dfrac{1 \text{ mL}}{50 \text{ mg}} = 0.4 \text{ mL}$

FIGURE 8-25

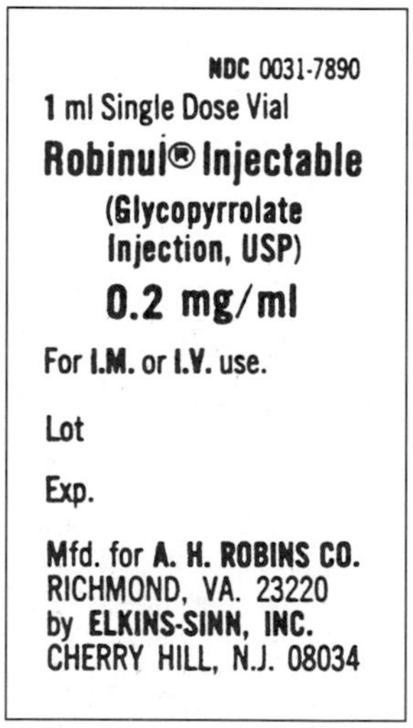

NDC 0031-7890

1 ml Single Dose Vial

Robinul® Injectable

(Glycopyrrolate
Injection, USP)

0.2 mg/ml

For I.M. or I.V. use.

Lot

Exp.

Mfd. for **A. H. ROBINS CO.**
RICHMOND, VA. 23220
by **ELKINS-SINN, INC.**
CHERRY HILL, N.J. 08034

EXAMPLE   Robinul 0.15 mg IM is ordered for the patient. On hand is a vial labeled: Robinul, (glycopyrrolate) 0.2 mg per mL (Figure 8-25). How many mL should be administered?

Equivalents: 0.2 mg = 1 mL

Conversion Equation:

$$0.15 \; \cancel{mg} \times \frac{1 \; mL}{0.2 \; \cancel{mg}} = 0.8 \; mL$$

FIGURE 8-26

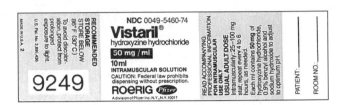

EXAMPLE   A patient is to receive Vistaril 35 mg IM. The medication comes in a vial labeled: Vistaril (hydroxyzine HCl) 50 mg per mL (Figure 8-26).

Equivalents: 50 mg = 1 mL

Conversion Equation:

$$35 \; \cancel{mg} \times \frac{1 \; mL}{50 \; \cancel{mg}} = 0.7 \; mL$$

PRACTICE

Calculating Dosages from Premixed Solutions

(**Note:** Use dimensional analysis and calculate the correct dosage to be administered per dose. Carry each answer to two decimal places and round to nearest tenth.

FIGURE 8-27

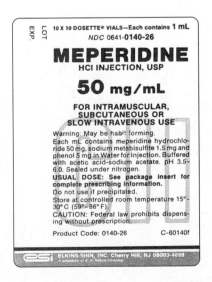

1. **Order:** Meperidine 30 mg IM
   Label: Figure 8-27
   How many milliliters should be administered?

FIGURE 8-28

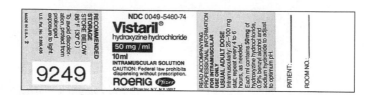

2. **Order:** Vistaril 75 mg IM
   Label: Figure 8-28. What is the generic name? _____
   How many milliliters should be administered?

FIGURE 8-29

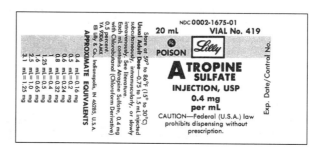

3. **Order:** Atropine Sulfate gr $\frac{1}{100}$ IM
   Label: Figure 8-29
   How many milliliters should be administered?

FIGURE 8-30

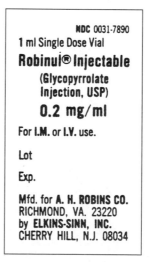

4. **Order:** Robinul 0.1 mg IM
   Label: Figure 8-30. What is the generic name? _____
   How many milliliters should be administered?

FIGURE 8-31

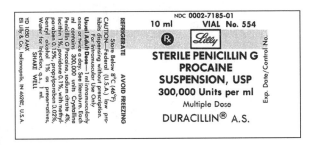

5. **Order:** Duracillin 450,000 U IM
   Label: Figure 8-31. What is the generic name? _____
   How many milliliters should be administered?

FIGURE 8-32

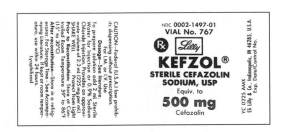

6. **Order:** Kefzol 135 mg IM
   Label: Figure 8-32. What is the generic name? _____
   How many milliliters should be administered?

FIGURE 8-33

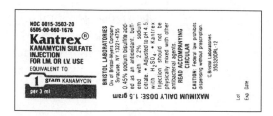

7. **Order:** Kantrex 150 mg IM
   Label: Figure 8-33 (3 mL = 1 g). What is the generic name? _____
   How many milliliters should be administered?

FIGURE 8-34

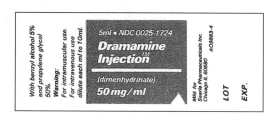

8. **Order:** Dramamine 35 mg IM
   Label: Figure 8-34. What is the generic name? _____
   How many milliliters should be administered?

FIGURE 8-35

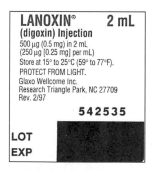

9. **Order:** Digoxin 0.125 mg IM
   Label: Figure 8-35. What is the trade name? _____
   How many milliliters should be administered?

FIGURE 8-36

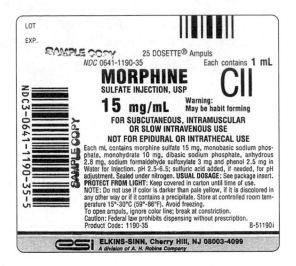

10. **Order:** Morphine Sulfate gr ⅛
    Label: Figure 8-36
    How many milliliters should be administered?

Determine the number of milliliters that should be administered in the following problems. (Carry all answers to two decimal places and round to the nearest tenth.)

11. **Order:** Phenobarbitol Sodium 100 mg IM
    Label: Phenobarbital Sodium 125 mg/2 mL

12. **Order:** Compazine 8 mg IM
    Label: Compazine (prochlorperazine) 10 mg/2 mL

13. **Order:** Valium 4 mg IM
    Label: Valium (diazepam) 5 mg/mL

14. **Order:** Vitamin K 20 mg IM
    Label: Vitamin K 25 mg/2.5 cc

15. **Order:** Lanoxin 0.25 mg IM
    Label: Lanoxin (digoxin) 500 μg/2 mL

16. **Order:** Cedilanid-D 0.6 mg IM
    Label: Cedilanid-D (deslanoside) 0.8 mg/4 mL

17. **Order:** Phenergan 40 mg IM
    Label: Phenergan (promethazine) 50 mg/mL

18. **Order:** Adrenalin Chloride 0.4 mg sc
    Label: Adrenalin Chloride (epinephrine HCl) 1 mg/2 mL

19. **Order:** Garamycin 60 mg IM
    Label: Garamycin (gentamicin sulfate) 40 mg/mL

20. **Order:** Fentanyl Citrate Injection 0.05 mg IM
    Label: Fentanyl Citrate Injection 100 mcg/2 mL

(**Note:** See Appendix G for answer key.)

Calculations Based on Body Weight

The method of calculating oral dosages based on body weight was described in Chapter 6. The method for calculating parenteral dosages is identical.

EXAMPLE

Order: Isoniazid Injection 5 mg/kg/day IM to an adult weighing 58 kg

Label: Isoniazid Injection 100 mg/mL

How many mL should be administered per dose?

$$58 \text{ kg} \times \frac{5 \text{ mg}}{1 \text{ kg}} \times \frac{1 \text{ mL}}{100 \text{ mg}} = 2.9 \text{ mL}$$

EXAMPLE

Order: Amikin 15 mg/kg/day IM in three divided doses to an adult weighing 155 lb

Label: Amikin (amikacin) 500 mg/2 mL

How many mL should be administered per dose?

$$155 \text{ lb} \times \frac{1 \text{ kg}}{2.2 \text{ lb}} \times \frac{15 \text{ mg}}{1 \text{ kg}} \times \frac{2 \text{ mL}}{500 \text{ mg}} = \frac{4.2 \text{ mL}}{3 \text{ doses}} = 1.4 \text{ mL/dose}$$

PRACTICE
IM Calculations Based on Body Weight

1. **Order:** Gentamicin Sulfate 3 mg/kg/24 hr IM in three divided doses to an adult weighing 77 kg
    Label: Gentamicin Sulfate 40 mg/mL
    How many mL should be administered per dose?

2. **Order:** Neomycin Sulfate 15 mg/kg/dose IM to an adult weighing 120 lb
    Label: Neomycin Sulfate 250 mg/mL
    How many mL should be administered per dose?

3. **Order:** Kanamycin Sulfate Injection 15 mg/kg/24 hr IM in three divided doses to an adult weighing 60 kg
    Label: Kanamycin Sulfate Injection 0.5 g/2 mL
    How many mL should be administered per dose?

4. **Order:** Bretylol 5 mg/kg IM in four divided doses to an adult weighing 190 lb
    Label: Bretylol (bretylium tosylate) 1 g/20 mL
    How many mL should be administered per dose?

5. **Order:** Nebcin 3 mg/kg/day IM in 3 divided doses to an adult weighing 80 kg
    Label: Nebcin (tobramycin sulfate) 80 mg/2 mL
    How many mL should be administered per dose?

6. **Order:** Benzquinamide 0.5 mg/kg/dose IM to an adult weighing 152 lb
   Label: Benzquinamide 25 mg/mL
   How many mL should be administered per dose?

7. **Order:** Amikacin Sulfate 15 mg/kg/day IM in two divided doses to an
   adult weighing 81.8 kg
   Label: Amikacin 500 mg/2 mL
   How many mL should be administered per dose?

8. **Order:** Kantrex Injection 15 mg/kg/day IM in four divided doses to an
   adult weighing 159 lb
   Label: Kantrex (kanamycin sulfate) Injection 1 g/3 mL
   How many mL should be administered per dose?

9. **Order:** Neobiotic 15 mg/kg/day IM in four divided doses to an adult
   weighing 78 kg
   Label: Neobiotic (neomycin sulfate) 250 mg/mL
   How many mL should be administered per dose?

10. **Order:** Nydrazid Injection 5 mg/kg/day IM in two divided doses to an
    adult weighing 128 lb
    Label: Nydrazid (isoniazid) Injection 100 mg/mL
    How many mL should be administered per dose?

(**Note:** See Appendix G for answer key.)

Units of Medication   Some drugs are measured in quantities called **units** (U). Unit quantities are frequently used for hormones, vitamins, antibiotics, antitoxins, and other biologicals. The value of a unit of drug is measured by the physiological effect a certain quantity will produce. Because the type of effect varies for each drug, there is no common definition for a unit. Vials of these drugs may vary in strength from a few units to millions of units per mL. Because this information is on the label, the quantity of solution to be administered can be calculated using these given equivalents.

Because many of the drugs dispensed in units are extremely potent, dosages are often very small, requiring use of special syringes that can measure small doses. For example, the tuberculin syringe can measure quantities as small as 0.01 mL. Clinical calculations involving medications that will be measured in a tuberculin syringe should be carried to three decimal places and rounded to the nearest hundredth in the following manner:

- If the digit in the thousandths place is less than 5, this digit is dropped.
- If the digit in the thousandths place is 5 or greater, the hundredths digit is increased by one. For example:

    0.256 mL; give 0.26 mL

    0.382 mL; give 0.38 mL

    0.615 mL; give 0.62 mL

The learner is reminded that insulin, which also is dispensed in units, should be measured only in an insulin syringe. Other medications that are ordered in larger quantities of units can be administered using a regular 2–3 cc syringe. Dimensional analysis is used to convert units to milliliters.

FIGURE 8-37

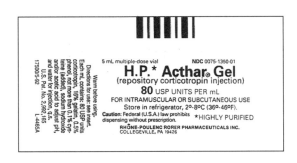

EXAMPLE   **Order:** H.P. Acthar Gel 50 U IM

Label: Figure 8-37

Dosage Strength: 80 U/mL

Conversion Equation:

$$50 \; \cancel{U} \times \frac{1 \text{ mL}}{80 \; \cancel{U}} = 0.63 \text{ mL}$$

Determine the number of milliliters that should be administered in the following problems. Carry all answers to two decimal places and round to the nearest tenth. Assume that dosages of less than 1 mL will be administered via tuberculin syringe; round appropriately.

FIGURE 8-38

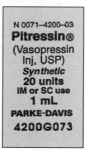

1. **Order:** Pitressin 8 U IM
   Label: Figure 8-38

FIGURE 8-39

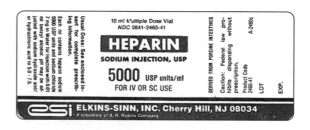

2. **Order:** Heparin Sodium Injection 3500 U sc
   Label: Figure 8-39

FIGURE 8-40

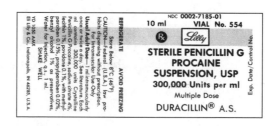

3. **Order:** Duracillin 500,00 U IM
   Label: Figure 8-40

FIGURE 8-41

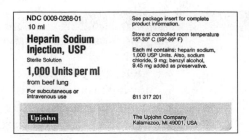

NDC 0009-0268-01
10 ml

**Heparin Sodium
Injection, USP**

Sterile Solution

1,000 Units per ml

from beef lung

For subcutaneous or
intravenous use

See package insert for complete
product information.

Store at controlled room temperature
15°-30° C (59°-86° F)

Each ml contains: heparin sodium,
1,000 USP Units. Also, sodium
chloride, 9 mg; benzyl alcohol,
9.45 mg added as preservative.

811 317 201

Upjohn

The Upjohn Company
Kalamazoo, MI 49001, USA

4. **Order:** Heparin 800 U sc
   Label: Figure 8-41

5. **Order:** Tetanus Immune Globulin 200 U IM
   Label: Tetanus Immune Globulin 250 U/mL

6. **Order:** Wycillin 450,000 U IM
   Label: Wycillin (penicillin G procaine) 600,000 U/mL

7. **Order:** Tetanus Antitoxin 2500 U IM
   Label: Tetanus Antitoxin 1500 U/mL

8. **Order:** A.C.T.H. "80" Injectable 90 U IM
   Label: A.C.T.H. "80" (corticotropin) Injectable 400 U/5 mL

9. **Order:** BCG Vaccine 800,000 U ID
   Label: BCG Vaccine 8,000,000 U/mL

10. **Order:** Vitamin A 15,000 U IM
    Label: Vitamin A 50,000 U/mL

(**Note:** See Appendix G for answer key.)

Reconstitution of Drugs in Powder Form

Some medications are dispensed in vials containing the drug in dry powder form for reconstitution. These drugs lose their potency a short time after being placed in solution; therefore, they are not reconstituted until they are ready to be used.

A sterile diluent, usually either water or 0.9% sodium chloride (normal saline), must be added according to directions on the label or the manufacturer's package insert. This diluent must be labeled *"Injection"* or *"For Injection,"* Figure 8-42. Because other diluents may be specified on the label or accompanying circular (insert), be sure to read this information carefully. It is important that only diluents designated in the directions be used for reconstitution, because these have been determined to be compatible with the drug or the IV solution to which the drug will be added. For example, if the directions state, "Reconstitute only with sterile water for injection," do *not* substitute bacteriostatic water for injection; this contains preservatives that may alter the pH of the reconstituted solution and/or the effectiveness of the drug.

After the diluent is added, the vial must be shaken well to dissolve the powdered drug, which can then be drawn up into a syringe and administered. In some instances, the dissolved drug will expand the total resulting volume of solution. This must be taken into account when identifying

FIGURE 8-42

| STERILE WATER FOR INJECTION, USP | 0.9% SODIUM CHLORIDE INJECTION, USP |
| For Drug Diluent Use Only | For Drug Diluent Use Only |

equivalents; for example, the addition of 2 mL of diluent to a measured amount of dry drug may result in a total volume exceeding 2 mL. Therefore, it is necessary to refer to either the label or the package insert to ascertain the correct dosage strength or concentration of the reconstituted solution and to use the correct dosage strength in your calculation.

The drug label or accompanying instructions state the amount of diluent that should be added to the container to result in a specific concentration of drug. In preparing a solution for intramuscular injection for adults or children, select the dilution that would provide the ordered dose in an amount not excessive: e.g., maximum is 3 mL per site for average size adult; 2 mL per site for child age 6–12; 1 mL per site for child age infant to 5 years. If a dose exceeds the maximum recommended volume, it should be divided and administered in two injections.

If the total amount of reconstituted medication is to be administered immediately (single dose vial), the expiration date need not be filled in, because the empty vial will be discarded. If the total amount of reconstituted medication is not to be administered immediately (multiple dose vial), the label or product insert will state how long the medication can be stored. This expiration date and/or time should then be written on the label, along with the initials of the person who reconstituted the drug.

Some reconstituted drugs can be frozen in individual doses and retain their potency for varying lengths of time. Once thawed, these drugs must be administered within a specified time period. Information regarding expiration date and/or time is found on the label or the package insert.

A Control (Lot) Number is stamped on the vial by the manufacturer. This refers to information regarding production and distribution of the drug.

FIGURE 8-43

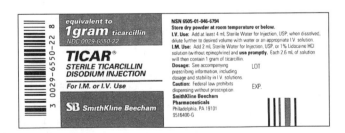

EXAMPLE

Order: Ticar (ticarcillin disodium) 500 mg IM

Label: Figure 8-43

a. What diluent(s) should be used? *Sterile Water for Injection USP* or *1% Lidocaine HCl Solution*

(without Epinephrine)

b. How many mL should be added to the vial? __2 mL__

c. What is the dosage strength of the prepared solution? __2.6 mL = 1 g__

d. How many mL should the patient receive?

$$500 \text{ mg} \times \frac{1 \text{ g}}{1000 \text{ mg}} \times \frac{2.6 \text{ mL}}{1 \text{ g}} = 1.3 \text{ mL}$$

Some drug labels will indicate that various amounts of diluent can be added to the vial to yield various concentrations of solution, Figure 8-44. After the drug has been reconstituted, the strength of the resulting solution should be indicated on the label (check, underscore, circle, or write in the appropriate dilution). In addition, the expiration date should be noted and initialed so that the drug will not be used beyond its expiration date.

FIGURE 8-44

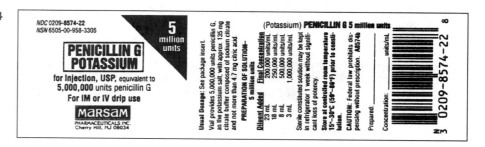

EXAMPLE

For each of the concentrations (dosage strength) listed on the label (Figure 8-44), how much diluent should be added to the vial and how much of the resulting solution would be administered to the patient if the order states: administer 600,000 U IM?

a. If 23 mL of diluent is added to the vial, the resulting solution will contain 200,000 U per mL.

Dosage Strength: 1 mL = 200,000 U

Conversation Equation:

$$600,000 \text{ U} \times \frac{1 \text{ mL}}{200,000 \text{ U}} = 3 \text{ mL}$$

b. If 18 mL of diluent is added to the vial, the resulting solution will contain 250,000 U per mL.

Dosage Strength: 1 mL = 250,000 U

Conversation Equation:

$$600,000 \text{ U} \times \frac{1 \text{ mL}}{250,000 \text{ U}} = 2.4 \text{ mL}$$

c. If 8 mL of diluent is added to the vial, the resulting solution will contain 500,000 U per mL.

Dosage Strength: 1 mL = 500,000 U

Conversation Equation:

$$600,000 \, \cancel{U} \times \frac{1 \text{ mL}}{500,000 \, \cancel{U}} = 1.2 \text{ mL}$$

d. If 3 mL of diluent is added to the vial, the resulting solution will contain 1,000,000 U per mL.

Dosage Strength: 1 mL = 1,000,000 U

Conversation Equation:

$$600,000 \, \cancel{U} \times \frac{1 \text{ mL}}{1,000,000 \, \cancel{U}} = 0.6 \text{ mL}$$

e. How long may the reconstituted solution be stored? <u>7 days</u>

f. Where should it be stored? <u>Refrigerator</u>

PRACTICE
Reconstitution of Drugs in Powder Form

FIGURE 8-45

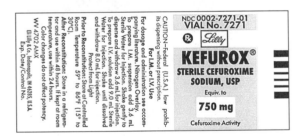

1. **Order:** Kefurox 500 mg IM
   Label: Figure 8-45; instructions for IM use. What is the generic name? _____

   a. How many mL should be added to the vial? _____

   b. How will you know what diluent to add? _____

   c. What is the dosage strength of the resulting solution? _____

   d. How many mL should the patient receive? _____

FIGURE 8-46

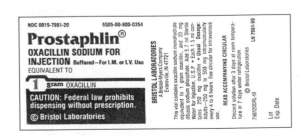

2. **Order:** Prostaphlin 300 mg IM
   Label: Figure 8-46; instructions for IM use. What is the generic name?
   _____

   a. What diluent should be used for reconstitution? _____

   b. How much diluent should be added to the vial? _____

   c. What is the dosage strength of the prepared solution? _____

   d. How many mL should the patient receive? _____

   e. What is the usual adult dose of this drug? _____

   f. Assume you reconstituted the drug at 10 A.M. on 9/16. What is the expiration time/date:

   - if you stored the vial at room temperature? _____

   - if you refrigerated the vial? _____

FIGURE 8-47

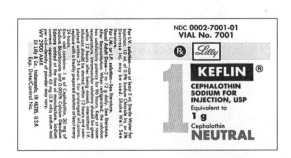

equivalent to
1gram ticarcillin
NDC 0029-6550-22

TICAR®
STERILE TICARCILLIN
DISODIUM INJECTION

For I.M. or I.V. Use

SB SmithKline Beecham

NSN 6505-01-046-6794
Store dry powder at room temperature or below.
I.V. Use: Add at least 4 mL Sterile Water for Injection, USP, when dissolved, dilute further to desired volume with water or an appropriate I.V. solution.
I.M. Use: Add 2 mL Sterile Water for Injection, USP, or 1% Lidocaine HCl solution (without epinephrine) and **use promptly.** Each 2.6 mL of solution will then contain 1 gram of ticarcillin.
Dosage: See accompanying prescribing information, including dosage and stability in I.V. solutions.
Caution: Federal law prohibits dispensing without prescription.
SmithKline Beecham
Pharmaceuticals
Philadelphia, PA 19101
9516400-G

LOT

EXP.

3. **Order:** Ticar 700 mg IM
   Label: Figure 8-47; instructions for IM use. What is the generic name?
   _____

   a. What diluent should be added to the vial? _____

   b. Assume you added 2 mL of diluent; what is the resulting dosage strength? _____

   c. How many mL should the patient receive? _____

   d. What other route can be used? _____

FIGURE 8-48

For I.V. solution—use at least 5 mL Sterile Water for Injection: 10 mL of 0.9% Sodium Chloride Inj. or 5% Dextrose Inj. may be used; Shake Well. See literature.
for I.M. or I.P. solution—See literature.
Usual Adult Dose—2 to 12 g daily. See literature.
After Reconstitution: When refrigerated, the solution has satisfactory potency for 96 hours, kept at room temperature, intramuscular solutions should be given within 12 hours after being mixed; intermittent I.V. infusions should be started within 12 hours and completed within 24 hours. For prolonged infusions, replace with a freshly prepared solution at least every 24 hours.
Each vial contains 1 g of Cephalothin, 30 mg of Sodium Bicarbonate and 0.005% Calcium Disodium Edetate added at the time of manufacture. Sodium content, approximately 65 mg (2.8 mEq) sodium ion per vial—density of powder may vary.
W 2900 AMX
Eli Lilly & Co. Indianapolis, IN 46285, U.S.A.
Exp. Date/Control No.

NDC 0002-7001-01
VIAL No. 7001

Rx *Lilly*

KEFLIN ®
CEPHALOTHIN
SODIUM FOR
INJECTION, USP
Equivalent to
1 g
Cephalothin

NEUTRAL

4. **Order:** Keflin 500 mg IM q 6 h
   Label: Figure 8-48; instructions for IM use: Each g should be diluted with 4 mL Sterile Water for Injection to yield a concentration of 0.5 g/2.2 mL. What is the generic name? _____

   a. What diluent should be added to the vial? _____

   b. How much diluent should be added to the vial? _____

   c. What is the dosage strength of the prepared solution? _____

   d. How many mL should the patient receive per dose? _____

   e. How many g would this patient receive over a 24 hr period? _____

   f. What is the usual adult dose of this drug? _____

   g. Assume you reconstituted the drug at 9 A.M. on 11/9. What is the expiration time/date if the solution is stored in the refrigerator? _____

   h. How soon after reconstitution must the medication be administered if it is not refrigerated? _____

FIGURE 8-49

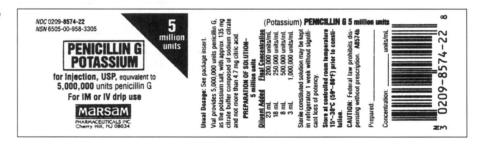

5. **Order:** Penicillin G Potassium 400,000 U IM qid
   For each concentration (dosage strength) listed on the label (Figure 8-49), calculate the number of mL the patient should receive.

   a. If 23 mL of diluent is added to the vial:

   Dosage Strength:

   Conversion Equation:

b. If 18 mL of diluent is added to the vial:

Dosage Strength:

Conversion Equation:

c. If 8 mL of diluent is added to the vial:

Dosage Strength:

Conversion Equation:

d. If 3 mL of diluent is added to the vial:

Dosage Strength:

Conversion Equation:

e. How long may the reconstituted solution be stored? _____

f. Where should the solution be stored? _____

Determine the number of milliliters that should be administered in the following problems. (Carry all answers to two decimal places and round to the nearest tenth.)

FIGURE 8-50

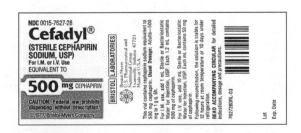

6. **Order:** Cephapirin Sodium 0.25 g IM
   Label: Figure 8-50

FIGURE 8-51

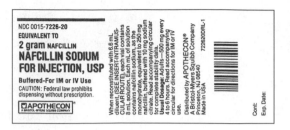

7. **Order:** Nafcillin Sodium 300 mg IM
   Label: Figure 8-51

FIGURE 8-52

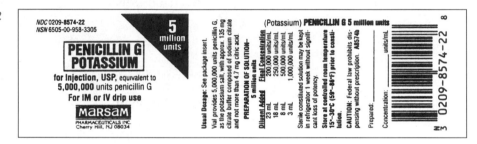

8. **Order:** Penicillin G Potassium 500,000 U IM
   Label: Figure 8-52
   Reconstitution: Add 23 mL of sterile diluent

9. **Order:** Ampicillin 150 mg IM
   Label: Ampicillin 500 mg—multiple dose vial
   Reconstitution: Add 1.8 mL of sterile diluent to yield 250 mg/mL

10. **Order:** Pipracil 800 mg IM
    Label: Pipracil (piperacillin sodium) 1 g powder form
    Reconstitution: Add 2 mL of sterile diluent to yield 1 g/2.5 mL

11. **Order:** Keflin 500 mg IM
    Label: Keflin (cephalothin) 1 g
    Reconstitution: Add 4 mL of sterile diluent to yield 0.5 g/2.2 mL

12. **Order:** Geopen 1 g IM
    Label: Geopen (carbexicillin disodium) 5 g
    Reconstitution: Add 7 mL of sterile diluent to yield 1 g/2 mL

13. **Order:** Polycillin-N 250 mg IM
    Label: Polycillin-N (ampicillin sodium) 1 g in dry form
    Reconstitution: Add 3.5 mL of sterile diluent to yield 250 mg/mL

14. **Order:** Unipen 400 mg IM
    Label: Unipen (nafcillin sodium) 1 g in powder form
    Reconstitution: Add 3.4 mL sterile water for injection to yield 1g/4mL

15. **Order:** Ampicillin 500 mg IM
    Label: Ampicillin 1 g/vial in dry form
    Reconstitution: Add 1.8 mL sterile water to yield 250 mg/mL

16. **Order:** Staphcillin 1.5 g IM
    Label: Staphcillin (methicillin sodium) 6 g vial in dry form
    Reconstitution: Add 8.6 mL of sterile normal saline to yield 500 mg/mL

17. **Order:** Streptomycin 1 g IM
    Label: Streptomycin 5 g in dry form
    Reconstitution: Add 9 mL of sterile water to yield 400 mg/mL

18. **Order:** Keflin 1 g IM
    Label: Keflin (cephalothin) 1 g in dry form
    Reconstitution: Add 4 mL of sterile water to yield 0.5 g/2.2 mL

19. **Order:** Penicillin G Sodium 300,000 U IM
    Label: Penicillin G Sodium 1,000,000 U/vial in dry form
    Reconstitution: Add 4.6 mL of sterile diluent to provide 200,000 U/mL

20. **Order:** Prostaphlin 150 mg IM
    Label: Prostaphlin (oxacillin sodium) 0.5 g/vial in dry form
    Reconstitution: Add 2.7 mL of sterile water to yield 250 mg/1.5 mL

(**Note:** See Appendix G for answer key.)

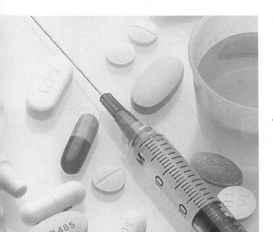

CHAPTER 9

Administration of Parenteral Medications

OBJECTIVES

Upon completion of this chapter you should be able to:

- Identify safe and suitable sites for intradermal, subcutaneous, and intramuscular injections, including boundaries and anatomical landmarks.

- Follow infection-control guidelines with respect to handling or manipulating needles and syringes.

- List the general rules for safe administration of parenteral medications: preparing, administering, and recording.

- Identify performance criteria related to administering drugs by subcutaneous and intramuscular routes, including variations when administering heparin and insulin.

- Read drug labels to differentiate various types of insulin.

Injection Sites and Techniques

A descriptive overview of injection sites and procedures follows, along with recommended guidelines for administration of parenteral medications. For detailed instruction on injection techniques, the learner is referred to a pharmacology or nursing text.

Intradermal Injection

Intradermal administration is the introduction of medication into the dermal layers of the skin. The needle penetrates the epidermis and enters the dermis. A very small amount of drug is given, usually for the purpose of skin testing. A 1 cc tuberculin syringe is used with a fine (25–26) gauge, $1/4''$–$5/8''$ needle. The medial surface of the forearm and the upper chest and back are the most commonly used sites, Figure 9-1. A very shallow angle of insertion, 10–15°, is used. The needle is inserted bevel up through the tautly held skin so that it is visible just beneath the surface and the medication is injected slowly until a small wheal is produced. Aspiration prior to injection is omitted. The needle is removed and the site wiped gently so as not to disperse the medication; the area is not massaged for the same reason. A bandage should not be applied and the patient should be instructed not to scratch or rub the site.

FIGURE 9-,1A,B
Intradermal injections

FRONT

BACK

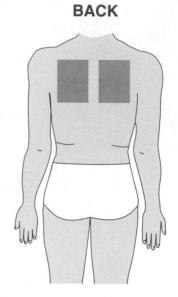

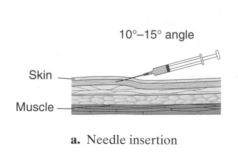

10°–15° angle

Skin

Muscle

a. Needle insertion

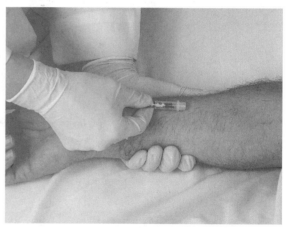

b. Holding skin

Subcutaneous Injection

Subcutaneous injection is the introduction of medication into the subcutaneous layer of connective and fatty tissue. Because this layer lies directly beneath the dermis, small amounts of solution are injected, usually not more than 2 mL in a site. A 1–3 mL syringe is used with a 25–28 gauge, ½″–⅝″ needle. Shorter or longer needles may be employed depending on the size and/or obesity of the recipient. When a ½″ needle is used, the needle is inserted at a 90° angle; with a ¾″–⅝″ needle, the angle of insertion is 45° bevel up, Figure 9-2. Subcutaneous injections may be administered at any site where there is an adequate layer of subcutaneous tissue. The most commonly used sites are: the upper outer arms, the anterior or lateral thighs, the abdomen from below the costal margins to the iliac crest (one and a half to two inches away from the umbilicus), the upper back below the scapulae, and the subcutaneous tissue over the dorsogluteal area. The areas over the deltoid and vastus lateralis or rectus femoris muscles often are used as long as the subcutaneous tissue can be bunched up so that

FIGURE 9-2A,B
Subcutaneous injections

FRONT

BACK

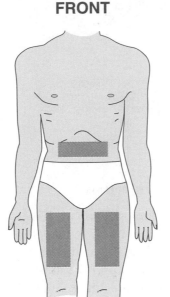

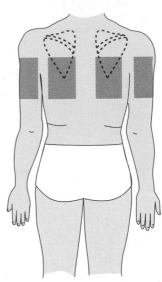

a. Subcutaneous sites

Angle of Insertion

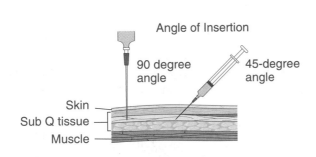

90 degree
angle

45-degree
angle

Skin
Sub Q tissue
Muscle

b. Bunch up tissue

the needle does not enter the muscle. When frequent subcutaneous injections are administered–such as daily insulin injections–a plan should be devised for rotating sites to promote absorption and avoid tissue fibrosis. Aspiration usually is performed prior to injection to avoid the possibility of intravascular injection, but there are exceptions to this rule. For example, persons with diabetes who self-administer insulin are no longer being taught to aspirate, for the purpose of facilitating this procedure. An inadvertent intravenous administration of insulin is not considered harmful. In the case of heparin, aspiration also is omitted, because the possibility of tissue damage with resulting subcutaneous bleeding. The nurse always should ascertain whether aspiration is required or contraindicated when administering subcutaneous injections.

FIGURE 9-3
Intramuscular injections

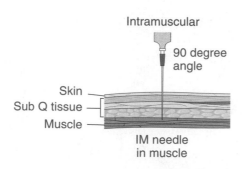

Intramuscular Injection

Intramuscular administration of medications is made through the skin and subcutaneous tissues into a muscle, Figure 9-3. Sites must be chosen with care to avoid damage to major nerves and blood vessels either by the needle or the medication. The most commonly used sites are the gluteal muscles. Also used are the deltoid, the vastus lateralis, and the rectus femoris. The sites should be rotated when the medication is irritating or repeated frequently.

The size of syringe and needle chosen depends on the amount and viscosity of medication to be given and the size and/or obesity of the recipient. For aqueous solutions, a 21 or 22 gauge, 1″–1½″ needle is usually suitable. For viscous or oily solutions, a 20 or 21 gauge needle of appropriate length is used. For both, a 90° angle of insertion is used.

It is necessary to aspirate prior to injection of the medication to avoid inadvertent intravenous injection. Following injection of most medications, the area is massaged gently to aid dispersion and absorption. The nurse always should ascertain the correct procedure regarding massage when intramuscular medications are administered.

Ventrogluteal Site   This site utilizes the ventral area of the gluteal muscles, specifically, the gluteus medius and minimus muscles below the iliac crest. These muscles can absorb up to 3 mL of solution per injection for an adult and 1–2 mL for children over the age of 1 year. This versatile site can be used with the patient in a lateral, supine, or prone position or—less desirable but possible—with the person standing or seated. Three anatomical landmarks are used to identify the site. The palm of the hand is placed on the greater trochanter of the femur, the index finger on the anterior superior iliac spine, and the middle finger abducted posteriorly along the iliac crest to form a V-shaped area. The injection site is in the center of the triangle between the index and middle fingers, Figure 9-4.

This is a safe injection site for both adults and for children over the age of 1 year. It is particularly useful in the case of small or emaciated persons, because the muscle layer is thick and easily accessible.

Dorsogluteal Site   The dorsogluteal site is located in the upper, outer quadrant of the buttock. Injection is made into the gluteus maximus muscle, which also can absorb up to 3 mL of solution for an adult. The patient may be positioned on one side or the other or on the abdomen with the toes pointed inward. The posterior iliac spine is palpated, as is the

FIGURE 9-4
Ventrogluteal site

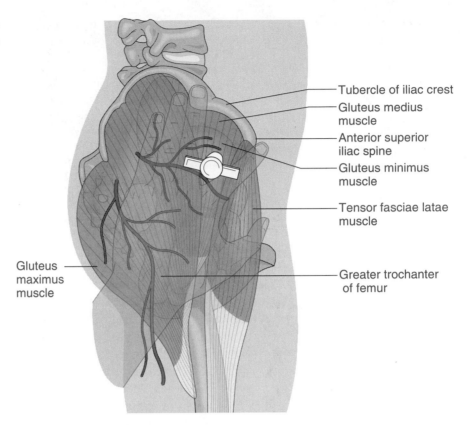

Tubercle of iliac crest

Gluteus medius
muscle

Anterior superior
iliac spine

Gluteus minimus
muscle

Tensor fasciae latae
muscle

Greater trochanter
of femur

Gluteus
maximus
muscle

greater trochanter of the femur, and an imaginary line is drawn between these two points. The injection site is lateral and superior to this line, Figure 9-5. The gluteal muscle is not used for infants, because it is small and poorly developed. The site may be used by the age of 3 years for children who have been walking at least a year, maximum volume 1–2 mL.

FIGURE 9-5 Dorsogluteal
site

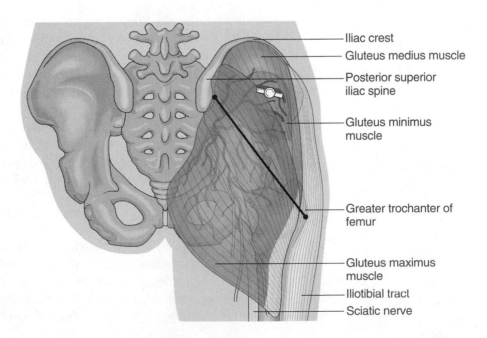

Iliac crest

Gluteus medius muscle

Posterior superior
iliac spine

Gluteus minimus
muscle

Greater trochanter of
femur

Gluteus maximus
muscle

Iliotibial tract

Sciatic nerve

FIGURE 9-6 Deltoid site

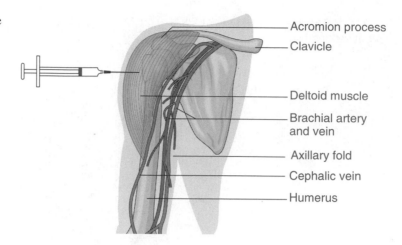

— Acromion process
— Clavicle
— Deltoid muscle
— Brachial artery and vein
— Axillary fold
— Cephalic vein
— Humerus

Deltoid Site The recommended site of injection into the deltoid muscle is into the thicker midportion of the muscle. This area is relatively small and is used when small amounts of solution are to be given, not exceeding 2 mL in adults. Because the deltoid muscle is very thin in infants and children, it is used only when very small amounts, not exceeding 0.5 mL, are to be given. The patient may be positioned on either side or sitting up. It is important that the arm hang loosely at the side when the patient is seated because this keeps the muscle relaxed. Holding the arm away from the body tenses the muscle and increases discomfort as well as impeding dispersion of the medication. The anatomical landmarks for identification of the deltoid site include the acromion process of the scapula and the axillary fold. The site is located at the center of the triangular area bounded superiorly by the acromion process and inferiorly by a line extending from the axillary fold across the lateral aspect of the arm, Figure 9-6.

Vastus Lateralis Site The vastus lateralis muscle is a commonly used injection site, because it is usually thick and well developed in both adults and children. The site can absorb up to 3 mL of solution, depending on the size of the individual. Smaller amounts should be administered to children. The patient may be in a lateral or supine position or sitting upright. The anatomical landmarks for identification of the site are the knee and the greater trochanter of the femur. Injection is made into the midportion of the muscle, located by measuring a hand's width above the knee and below the trochanter. The muscle extends from the midanterior to midlateral thigh between the two bony landmarks, Figure 9-7.

Rectus Femoris Site The rectus femoris muscle, on the anterior aspect of the thigh, can be used for intramuscular injections of up to 3 mL and is especially accessible for individuals who self-administer their injections. The patient assumes a sitting or lying position and the injection site is in the lateral midportion of the anterior thigh. The medial aspect of the thigh should be avoided, Figure 9-8. This site may be used for children and infants, no more than 1–2 mL depending on age and size.

FIGURE 9-7 Vastus lateralis site

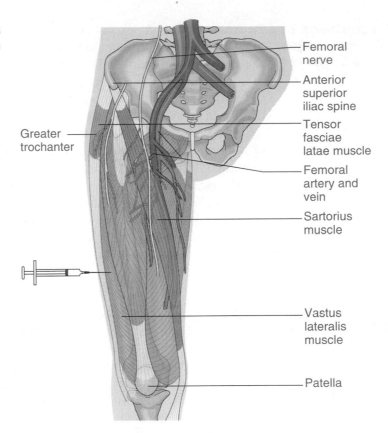

Femoral nerve

Anterior superior iliac spine

Tensor fasciae latae muscle

Femoral artery and vein

Sartorius muscle

Greater trochanter

Vastus lateralis muscle

Patella

FIGURE 9-8 Rectus femoris site

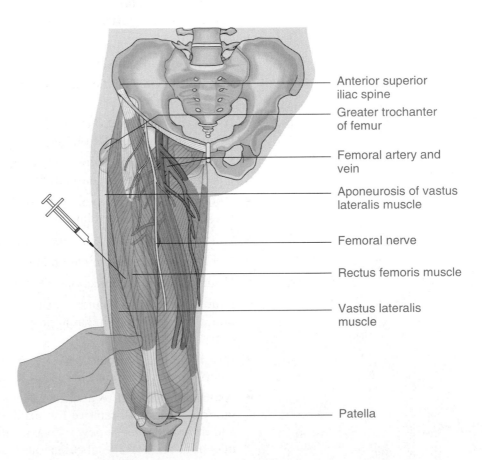

Anterior superior iliac spine

Greater trochanter of femur

Femoral artery and vein

Aponeurosis of vastus lateralis muscle

Femoral nerve

Rectus femoris muscle

Vastus lateralis muscle

Patella

Precautions in Handling Needles and Syringes

Because of the risk associated with contacting blood contaminated with microorganisms, personnel must use special precautions when handling all used needles and syringes. It is recommended that a glove be placed on the nondominant hand (i.e., the hand that comes into contact with the patient) when any injection is administered. In addition, because of the danger of needle-stick injuries, used needles should not be recapped, bent, or broken following injection. They should not be removed from disposable syringes or otherwise manipulated by hand. All used needles and syringes should immediately be discarded into puncture-resistant containers. Personnel should ascertain agency policy with regard to handling and disposing of syringes and needles, and they should follow these guidelines meticulously. Any time gloves are worn when handling needles and syringes, hands should be washed thoroughly immediately after gloves are removed, even if the gloves appear to be intact.

Administration of Parenteral Medications

The general rules for administration of medications, which were listed in Chapter 7, also apply here. Because of the additional potential for harm to the patient when medications are given parenterally, accuracy and care in preparing and administering these drugs assumes critical proportions. Precise identification of sites and proper techniques of administration cannot be overemphasized. Principles of safety, comfort, and effective intervention are equally important.

In addition to the rules in Chapter 7, specific recommendations for administration of intradermal, subcutaneous, and intramuscular injections include:

- Select a sterile syringe and needle of the appropriate size and length.
- Mix solution in vial, if necessary, by rotating between palms or shaking gently.
- If irritating medications are being administered, it is desirable to change the needle after obtaining the correct dose.
- Carefully select and identify injection sites by fully exposing area and palpating anatomical landmarks.
- Rotate injection sites as appropriate for repeated injections. A chart or diagram for rotation of injection sites is often desirable.
- Obtain assistance as necessary if patient needs to be restrained.
- Place glove on nondominant hand.
- Cleanse skin at the injection site with an antiseptic wipe.
- Hold syringe in one hand; with the other hand bunch or hold the skin taut at the injection site, as appropriate for type of injection and angle of insertion.
- Insert the needle about seven-eighths of its length, thus preventing complete disappearance in case of breakage.
- Aspirate for blood to avoid an accidental intravascular injection. If blood is aspirated, remove the needle, obtain a new needle, syringe, and dose and select a new site. Aspiration is omitted with intradermal injections and certain subcutaneous medications (i.e., insulin, heparin).

- Inject the medication into the tissue with slow, steady pressure.

- For IM injection, place the antiseptic wipe adjacent to the needle, apply reverse pressure, and quickly withdraw the needle, immediately making slight pressure over the site with the wipe.

- For subcutaneous injection: (longer needle, 45° angle, bevel up), lay the antiseptic wipe over the injection site without exerting pressure on the needle, quickly remove the needle, and then apply pressure over the site; shorter needle, 90° angle, proceed as in IM injection above.

- Gently massage the injection site with an antiseptic wipe to increase the rate of dispersion and absorption. Avoid massage with intradermal, insulin, heparin, or Z-track.

- Discard used syringe and needle (without recapping) into puncture-resistant container.

The learner may find the following checklist a helpful guide for the administration of parenteral medications.

Performance Criteria: Administration of Injections

	S	U	Comments
A. Preparing the medication			
1. Obtains medication MAR to confirm medication order regarding dose, route, and time of administration			
2. Checks for any known allergies			
3. Washes hands			
4. Selects appropriate size syringe and needle			
a) Intradermal injection: 1 cc tuberculin syringe with 25–27 gauge, ¼″ to ⅝″ needle			
b) Subcutaneous injection: 1–3 cc syringe with 25–28 gauge, ½″ to ⅝″ needle			
c) Intramuscular injection: 1–3 cc syringe with 20–22 gauge, 1″ to 1½″ needle			
5. Obtains correct medication (vial, ampule, or cartridge)			
6. Checks medication label against MAR			
7. Checks for expiration date of medication			

Continues

	S	U	Comments
8. Withdraws medication into syringe			
a) *Vial:* **1.** cleanses stopper with antiseptic wipe			
2. injects air into vial equal to amount of medication to be withdrawn			
3. withdraws accurate dosage of medication, changes needle where appropriate			
b) *Glass Ampule:* **1.** wraps ampule in gauze or antiseptic wipe			
2. snaps off top of ampule			
3. places needle into open ampule and withdraws required dosage			
c) *Double Vial Technique:* (Mixing two medications in one syringe) **1.** cleanses stoppers on both vials with antiseptic wipe			
2. placing first vial on a flat surface, injects air into air space equal to the desired dose			
3. injects air into second vial equal to the desired dose and then withdraws this amount of medication			
4. recleanses top of first vial, reinserts needle, and withdraws desired dose, being careful not to inject any medication from second vial			
5. returns or disposes of drug container properly			

	S	U	Comments
6. rechecks labels against the MAR			
d) *Prefilled cartridge:* **1.** inserts into cartridge holder			
2. ejects excess air			

B. Administering the injection
   1. *Intradermal*
     a) Identifies the correct patient			

b) Selects correct site —ventral forearm			
—upper chest area			
—subscapular area			
c) Places glove on nondominant hand			
d) Cleanses site with antiseptic wipe and allows to dry			
e) Spreads the site to hold tissue taut			
f) Positions syringe so needle is at 10° to 15° angle to the patient's skin; bevel up			
g) Inserts needle ⅛″ below skin's surface with point visible through skin			
h) Injects medication slowly until wheal forms			
i) Withdraws needle, blots gently with antiseptic wipe, avoiding massage			
j) Places used syringe and needle (without recapping) into puncture-resistant container			
2. *Subcutaneous* **a)** Identifies correct patient			
b) Provides privacy			

Continues

	S	U	Comments
c) Selects correct site			
—outer aspects of upper arms			
—anterior and outer aspects of thighs			
—abdomen, above iliac crests (1½–2″ away from umbilicus)			
—subscapular region of back			
—dorso-ventrogluteal area			
d) Places glove on nondominant hand			
e) Cleanses site with antiseptic wipe			
f) Grasps skin between thumb and forefinger to elevate subcutaneous tissue			
g) Inserts ½″ needle at 90° angle to skin and ⅝″ needle at 45° angle with bevel up			
h) Releases skin and grasps hub of syringe to stabilize needle			
i) Aspirates for blood, keeping needle and syringe steady. If blood appears, withdraws needle, discards medication, obtains new syringe, needle, and dose, and selects new site			
j) Injects medication slowly			
k) Places antiseptic wipe over (45°) or adjacent to (90°) the needle without applying pressure			
l) Removes needle quickly and immediately applies pressure with antiseptic wipe			
m) Massages site gently, unless contraindicated			

	S	U	Comments
n) Discards used syringe and needle (without recapping) into puncture-resistant container			
3. *Intramuscular*			
a) Identifies correct patient			
b) Provides privacy			
c) Selects correct site —ventrogluteal			
—dorsogluteal			
—deltoid			
—vastus lateralis			
—rectus femoris			
d) Places glove on nondominant hand			
e) Positions patient and exposes site			
f) Cleanses site with antiseptic wipe			
g) Stretches skin taut at injection site			
h) Quickly injects needle at 90° angle, using a dartlike thrust			
i) Releases stretched skin and grasps hub of syringe to stabilize needle			
j) Aspirates for blood, keeping needle and syringe steady. If blood appears, withdraws needle, discards medication, obtains new syringe, needle, and dose, and selects a new site			
k) Injects medication slowly			
l) Places antiseptic wipe adjacent to site			

Continues

	S	U	Comments
m) Withdraws needle quickly and immediately applies antiseptic wipe			
n) Massages site gently, unless contraindicated			
o) Discards used syringe and needle (without recapping) into puncture-resistant container			
C. Following injection **1.** Leaves patient comfortable			
2. Disposes of equipment according to hospital policy			
3. Records accurately			
D. Maintains principles of asepsis throughout the procedure			
E. Maintains principles of patient safety and comfort throughout the procedure			

S—Satisfactory   U—Unsatisfactory   Evaluator _____

Variation of Parenteral Injection Techniques: IM

Z-Track

This is a method of administering a deep intramuscular injection to prevent seepage of medication along the needle track. The method is used when any medication that is irritating or a substance that stains such as iron is given, because it is more effective in sealing medication within the desired site than the customary (usual) intramuscular injection technique. Figure 9-9 illustrates the technique of Z-track injection.

FIGURE 9-9 The Z-track technique for deep intramuscular injection (Courtesy of Reiss and Evans, *Pharmacological Aspects of Nursing Care*, 5th ed. Copyright 1996 by Delmar Publishers, Inc. NY)

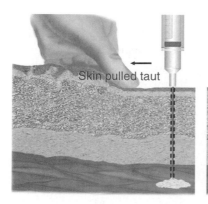
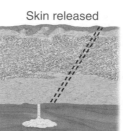

Skin pulled taut   Skin released

It is important to select a deep site in a large muscle, preferably the dorsogluteal site. See Figure 9-9. It is also important to apply a new needle after obtaining the desired dose to prevent depositing medication in the subcutaneous tissues as the needle is inserted into the muscle. In addition, a 0.5 mL air lock is used to clear the needle of medication after injection and to help prevent leakage or tracking. Therefore, after the correct dosage is obtained, 0.5 mL of air is drawn into the syringe to provide the desired air lock following injection of the medication.

Performance Criteria: Z-Track Method—Deep Intramuscular Injection

(**Note:** Follows usual procedure for intramuscular injection with the following modifications.)

	S	U	Comments
1. Selects appropriate size syringe with suitable needle for withdrawing medication. (This needle will be discarded.)			
2. After obtaining medication, pulls back plunger to add 0.5 mL air lock			
3. Replaces needle with sterile needle, 20 or 21 gauge, 1¼″–1½″ long (for iron—19 or 20 gauge, 2″–3″ long)			
4. Uses dorsogluteal site (this is the only acceptable site)			
5. Places glove on nondominant hand			
6. Displaces skin firmly to one side, then cleanses selected site with antiseptic wipe			
7. Inserts needle at 90° angle			
8. While maintaining retracted skin, aspirates for blood, then injects medication slowly			
9. Waits 10 seconds (still maintaining skin retraction)			
10. Withdraws needle quickly, simultaneously releasing retracted skin			
11. Does *NOT* massage site			

Continues

	S	U	**Comments**
12. Discards used syringe and needle (without recapping) into puncture-resistant container			
13. Records location of injection site (rotates site)			

S—Satisfactory   U—Unsatisfactory   Evaluator _____

In the Z-track technique, the skin and subcutaneous tissues are displaced to one side, resulting in a shift of tissue layers out of normal alignment (see Figure 9-9). The needle is inserted directly into the muscle layer and the medication is injected slowly while tissue displacement is maintained. It is therefore necessary to aspirate and hold the syringe with the same hand. A period of 10 seconds is allowed to elapse before needle removal to ensure adequate dispersion. When the needle is removed, the tissues are quickly released and return to their normal position, leaving a Z-shaped channel that prevents seepage and tracking. The site is not massaged.

The checklist on pp. 000–000 may be used as a guide for the Z-track variation.

Variation of Parenteral Injection Techniques: SC

Heparin Injection

Subcutaneous injection of heparin requires special modifications in technique to cause as little trauma as possible to the tissues at the injection site. The purpose is to prevent or minimize bleeding caused by the anticoagulant properties of this drug. To avoid inadvertent intramuscular injection, it is important to select a short needle and a site with adequate subcutaneous tissue. Separate needles should be used for obtaining and injecting the heparin. Sites on the abdomen above the level of the anterior iliac spines are most commonly used, Figure 9-10. It is important to rotate sites and to select sites free from bruising or scarring and at least 2″ away from the umbilicus. Gentle cleansing of the skin helps prevent trauma, as does omission of aspiration and massage. The patient also should be reminded not to rub the site. Application of an icebag following injection may prevent ecchymosis.

The following checklist may be used as a guide for the heparin injection.

FIGURE 9-10   Heparin sites

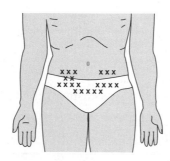

Performance Criteria: Administration of Heparin

(**Note:** Follows usual procedure for subcutaneous injection with the following modifications.)

	S	U	Comments
1. Selects appropriate size syringe with 25–27 gauge needle, $\frac{1}{2}''$–$\frac{5}{8}''$ long plus second sterile needle for injection			
2. Obtains correct dose and changes needle			
3. Selects correct site: abdomen, above the anterior iliac spines and 2″ away from umbilicus, scars, or ecchymoses			
4. Places glove on nondominant hand			
5. Gently bunches a well-defined roll of tissue without pinching			
6. Wipes site with antiseptic wipe (avoids rubbing)			
7. While maintaining roll, inserts needle at a 90° angle into subcutaneous fatty tissue. Does *NOT* aspirate for blood. While still maintaining roll of tissue and keeping needle steady, slowly injects medication			
8. Withdraws needle in same direction of insertion while simultaneously releasing tissue roll			
9. Holds antiseptic wipe at injection site for $\frac{1}{2}$–1 minute. Does *NOT* massage site			
10. Discards used syringe and needle (without recapping) into puncture-resistant container			
11. Records location of injection site (rotates injection sites)			

S—Satisfactory   U—Unsatisfactory   Evaluator _____

Insulin Preparations   Persons who have diabetes caused by insulin-secretion deficiency may be treated by regular (daily or more often) injections of manufactured insulin. Synthetic human insulin is most widely used in this country. Other sources of manufactured insulin are: pork pancreas, beef pancreas, or a combination of the two. Because allergic reactions are possible, alternative forms of insulin may be prescribed. If the source is identified in the insulin order, it is essential that the correct bottle be selected, Figure 9-11.

Insulins differ as to time of onset, peak of activity, and duration of action. These characteristics are controlled by adding zinc and/or protamine to regular (fast-acting) insulin to produce either intermediate or long-acting effects. These extended-action products are called *modified* insulins and are designated by the letters S, L, N, P, and U.

Regular insulin is a clear solution designated by the letter R on the bottle. An example is shown in Figure 9-11. It can be administered subcutaneously or intravenously. It is important to remember that regular insulin is the *only type of insulin* that can be administered intravenously.

Due to the suspension of zinc and/or protamine, modified insulin is cloudy, and *only* can be administered subcutaneously. Figure 9-12 shows two examples.

A combination of regular and modified insulins often is ordered to provide for both rapid and prolonged action. One such combination, currently on the market, contains 70% modified and 30% regular insulins premixed, Figure 9-13. These insulin mixtures are convenient to use when the prescribed dose is identical to the mixture available. However, in many

FIGURE 9-11   Regular insulin

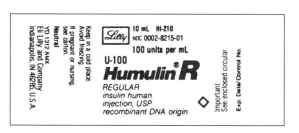

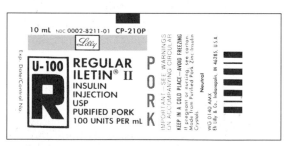

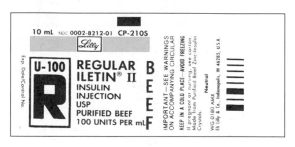

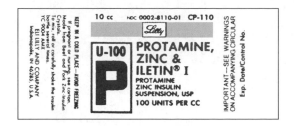

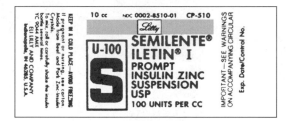

FIGURE 9-12   Modified insulin

FIGURE 9-13   Pre-mixed insulin

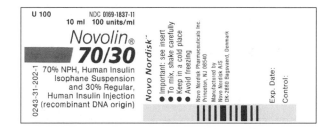

instances this is not the case. If an identical combination is not available, the ordered insulin dosages may be administered separately or mixed in one syringe for administration. In mixing two different types of insulin in one syringe, it is important that no modified insulin be introduced into the bottle of regular insulin. Therefore, when mixing two types of insulin in one syringe, the regular insulin (clear) should be drawn up first and the modified insulin (cloudy) second. (See Procedure for Mixing Insulins, page 000.) Because mixtures of insulin remain stable for only a few minutes, it is important to administer these injections immediately after mixing them. Regardless of whether regular, modified, or mixed insulins are ordered, it is essential that the correct type be selected and that the exact prescribed amount be administered.

Insulin preparations should be stored in a cold place, preferably refrigerated, but not frozen. Insulin currently in use may be stored unrefrigerated, as long as it is kept as cool as possible and away from sunlight or direct heat. Insulin kept at room temperature will last a month or so. Label date should be checked and no insulin should be used beyond its expiration date.

PRACTICE
Reading Insulin Labels

From Figure 9-14, select the correct bottle (by letter) and answer the questions relating to the insulin order.

1. What is the concentration of each of the insulin preparations shown?

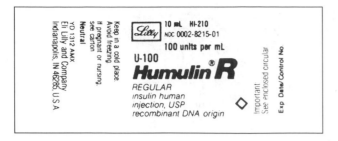

a.

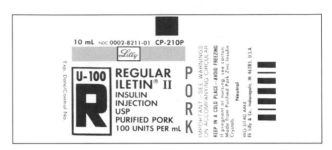

b.

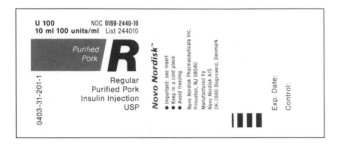

c.

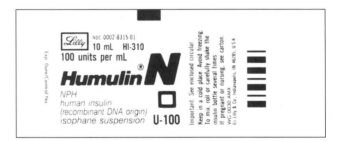

d.

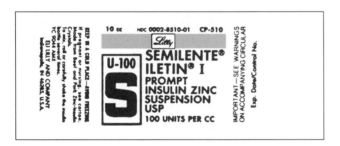

e.

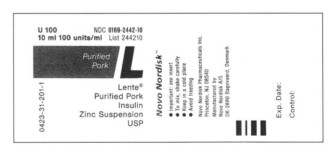

f.

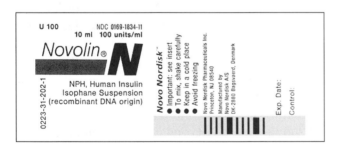

g.

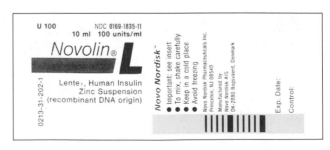

h.

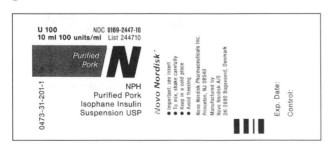

i.

j.

Note: On the Lilly label, Iletin I means the source is mixed beef and pork, Iletin II means the source is pure beef or pure pork.

FIGURE 9-14   Fast-acting, intermediate and long-acting insulin.

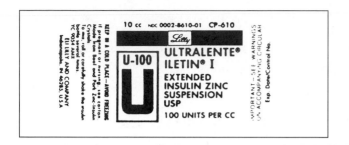

k.

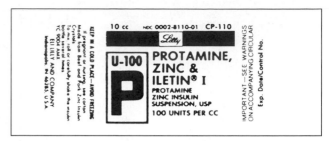

l.

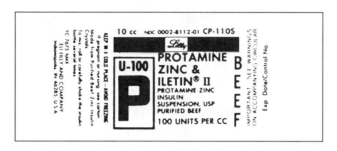

m.

FIGURE 9-14   Fast-acting, intermediate and long-acting insulins

2. Identify the two manufacturers represented. _____

3. Select by letter:

   ■ All of the varieties of human (synthetic) insulin pictured. _____

   ■ All of the varieties of NPH insulin pictured. _____

   ■ Two labels identifying insulin modified with both protamine and zinc. _____

   ■ A regular insulin prepared from pork. _____

   ■ A semilente insulin prepared from beef. _____

   ■ All the preparations from a mixed (beef/pork) source. _____

4. What letter appears on the label for:

   ■ Regular Insulin _____

   ■ Semilente Insulin _____

   ■ NPH Insulin _____

   ■ Lente Insulin _____

   ■ Ultralente Insulin _____

   ■ Protamine, Zinc Insulin _____

5. Prepare the following doses of insulin for administration. You have available a 1 cc, U-100 syringe. Select (by letter) the correct medication label from Figure 9-14.

   a. Order: Humulin R Insulin 24 units sc

       1. **Label:** _____

       2. How much insulin would you withdraw? _____ U

   b. Order: Lente (Pork) Insulin 45 units sc

       1. **Label:** _____

       2. How much insulin would you withdraw? _____ U

   c. Order: Regular Insulin 10 units and Protamine Zinc (Beef) Insulin 38 units sc

       1. **Labels:** _____

       2. Which insulin would be drawn up first? _____

       3. What is the total amount of insulin mixed in the syringe? _____ units

   d. Order: Regular (Purified Pork) Insulin 24 units and Lente (Pork) Insulin 42 units sc

       1. **Labels:** _____

       2. Which insulin would be drawn up last?_____

       3. What is the total amount of insulin mixed in the syringe? _____ units

---

(**Note:** See Appendix G for answer key.)

Insulin Administration

Insulin is ordered and measured in USP units. Almost universally used is the concentration of 100 units per milliliter, designated on the bottle as U-100 insulin, Figure 9-15. This means that 1 mL of the product contains 100 units of insulin. Insulin syringes for this strength are available in two sizes, a 1 cc size that measures up to 100 units (Figure 9-16) and a 0.5 cc size that measures up to 50 units; these are referred to commonly as U-100 syringes. They usually are prepackaged with a 27 or 28 gauge, ½″ needle. Use of the unit-calibrated insulin syringe eliminates the need for calculation, because it is only necessary to draw up the ordered number of units. Neither a tuberculin syringe nor a 2–3 mL syringe gives precise enough measurement; these never should be used for insulin.

    Insulin is also available in U-500 concentrations; one mL containing 500 units of insulin. This strength also requires a specially calibrated syringe

FIGURE 9-15 U-100 Insulin

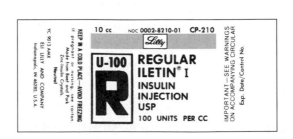

FIGURE 9-16   Insulin
                syringes

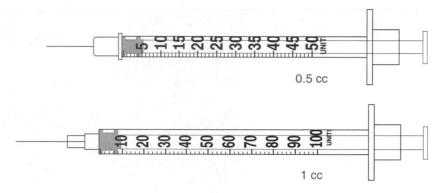

0.5 cc

1 cc

for measuring. U-500 insulin is a concentration of regular insulin that can be administered by either subcutaneous or intramuscular routes. The intravenous route is not recommended.

It is essential that the calibrations of the syringe match the concentration of the insulin, that is, the number of units per milliliter. The nurse must be careful to ascertain the strength of the insulin being administered and use the correctly calibrated syringe.

Insulin Injection

Because most persons who require insulin injections are eventually taught to self-administer this hormone, nurses must be alert to the learning needs of these patients and must teach and reinforce correct principles of insulin administration.

Because the insulin injection is repeated daily or more often, it is essential to rotate injection sites to prevent tissue damage or complications such as atrophy, thickening, or scarring, all of which can interfere with proper absorption. Patients should be taught to alternate sites using a site selection plan that will help ensure proper rotation.

Patients may also need to learn how to mix combinations of insulin preparations in one syringe. It is important to stress that the short-acting (regular) insulin be withdrawn prior to withdrawal of long-acting (modified) insulin. It is essential that any air bubbles be eliminated from the syringe when obtaining the dose of insulin to have an accurate amount. The step for aspirating for blood prior to injection is omitted in teaching self-administration of insulin, because it is difficult for patients to do this one-handed.

In addition to the insulin syringe and needle, other insulin injection devices are currently available that offer accuracy, convenience, and versatility for persons who self-administer their insulin. One such example, shown in Figure 9-17, can be easily carried about and facilitates daily single or multiple injections of premixed insulin (Figure 9-18), thereby greatly simplifying the procedure and routine of insulin self-administration.

Any area of subcutaneous tissue can be used for insulin administration. Diabetic patients most frequently use the abdomen and thighs for self-administration sites. When insulin is administered by other persons, the upper arms and gluteal areas can be used, Figure 9-19.

FIGURE 9-17 Insulin injection system for self-administration

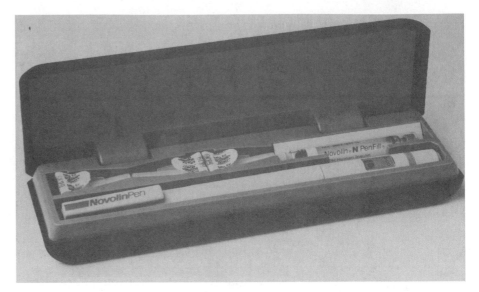

NDC 0169-0017-71 *Novo Nordisk*	NDC 0169-0017-71 *Novo Nordisk*	NDC 0169-0017-71 *Novo Nordisk*
List 001771	List 001771	List 001771
*Novolin **70/30** Prefilled.*	*Novolin **70/30** Prefilled.*	*Novolin **70/30** Prefilled.*
70% NPH, Human Insulin Isophane Suspension and 30% Regular, Human Insulin Injection (recombinant DNA origin)	70% NPH, Human Insulin Isophane Suspension and 30% Regular, Human Insulin Injection (recombinant DNA origin)	70% NPH, Human Insulin Isophane Suspension and 30% Regular, Human Insulin Injection (recombinant DNA origin)
100 units/ml 1.5 ml Prefilled Insulin Syringe	100 units/ml 1.5 ml Prefilled Insulin Syringe	100 units/ml 1.5 ml Prefilled Insulin Syringe
Novo Nordisk Pharmaceuticals Inc. Princeton, NJ 08540	Novo Nordisk Pharmaceuticals Inc. Princeton, NJ 08540	Novo Nordisk Pharmaceuticals Inc. Princeton, NJ 08540
9842-31-201-1 Exp. Date: Control:	9842-31-201-1 Exp. Date: Control:	9842-31-201-1 Exp. Date: Control:

FIGURE 9-18 Pre-mixed insulin

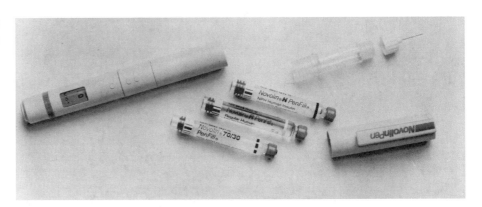

NDC 0169-1837-17	NDC 0169-1833-17	NDC 0169-1834-17
*Novolin® **70/30** PenFill®*	*Novolin® **R** PenFill®*	*Novolin® **N** PenFill.*
70% NPH, Human Insulin Isophane Suspension and 30% Regular, Human Insulin Injection (r-DNA origin)	Regular, Human Insulin Injection (r-DNA origin)	NPH, Human Insulin Isophane Suspension (r-DNA origin)
1.5 ml 100 units/ml	100 units/ml 1.5 ml	100 units/ml 1.5 ml
For information contact: Novo Nordisk Pharmaceuticals Inc. Princeton, NJ 08540	For information contact: Novo Nordisk Pharmaceuticals Inc. Princeton, NJ 08540	For information contact: Novo Nordisk Pharmaceuticals Inc. Princeton, NJ 08540
0245-31-201-1	0205-31-201-1	0225-31-201-1

FIGURE 9-19 Insulin injection sites and rotation patterns

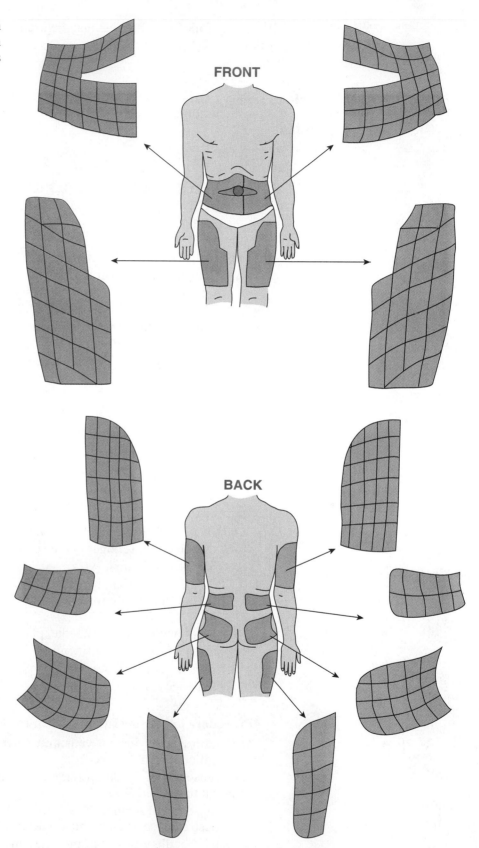

The following checklist may be used as a guide for insulin administration.

Performance Criteria: Administration of Insulin

(**Note:** Follows usual procedure for subcutaneous injection with the following modifications.)

	S	U	Comments
1. Selects appropriate size (0.3, 0.5 or 1 cc) insulin syringe with ½″ needle			
2. Rolls vial of modified insulin between hands to mix (avoids shaking)			
*3. When mixing two insulins in one syringe, withdraws regular insulin into syringe first, then modified insulin			
4. Selects correct site according to previously established plan for rotation of sites			
5. Places glove on nondominant hand			
6. Pinches cleansed site between thumb and forefinger and inserts needle at 90° angle			
7. Does not aspirate for blood			
8. Upon withdrawal of needle, places antiseptic wipe over site and presses lightly. Does *NOT* massage			

*Procedure for Mixing Insulins (clear to cloudy)
1. Obtain correct insulin vials and correct insulin syringe/needle. Roll modified insulin to mix.
2. Cleanse top of modified (cloudy) insulin and inject air into air space equal to desired dose
3. Cleanse top of regular (clear) insulin and inject air into air space equal to desired dose, then withdraw desired dose of regular insulin
4. Insert needle into vial of modified insulin and withdraw desired dose, being careful not to introduce any regular insulin into vial
5. Gently rotate syringe to mix insulins

	S	U	Comments
9. Discards used syringe and needle (without recapping) into puncture-resistant container			
10. Records administration on diabetic record as well as on medication record and/or site selection plan			

S—Satisfactory   U—Unsatisfactory   Evaluator _____

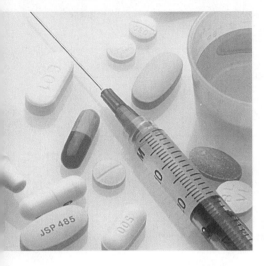

CHAPTER 10

Calculations of Intravenous Medications and Solutions

OBJECTIVES

Upon completion of this chapter you should be able to:

- Identify equipment used in the administration of intravenous medications and solutions, including types of needles and cannulas, infusion sets, and solution containers.

- Describe the various methods by which intravenous medications/solutions may be administered: continuous IV drip, IV piggyback, volume control set, heparin lock, central venous catheter, and IV bolus.

- Read drug labels to obtain necessary information for administration of IV medications and solutions.

- Demonstrate knowledge of the appropriate method for rounding off when calculating IV flow rates.

- Apply dimensional analysis to clinical calculations involving medications administered intravenously.

- Identify nursing responsibilities in relation to assessing and adjusting intravenous infusions.

Intravenous Injections and Infusions

Intravenous administration refers to the injection or infusion of medications and fluids into a vein. It is another example of parenteral administration. Because the medication enters the circulation directly, the effect of drugs given intravenously is immediate. The abbreviation IV is used for these medication orders.

This unit deals with equipment and solutions used in administering IVs, reading labels and adding medications, and calculating IV drug dosages.

Equipment

Needles, Catheters, and Cannulas

Generally, a needle with a plastic catheter attached is used to administer intravenous fluids. After venipuncture, the catheter is threaded into the vein and remains in place when the needle is withdrawn. This combination needle/catheter is called a cannula. A plastic catheter that passes through the needle bore (inside-the-needle catheter) is called an intracath; one that covers the needle (over-the-needle catheter) is called an angiocath. Intravenous catheters vary in length from $1\frac{1}{4}''$ to $36''$ and in diameter from 12G to 22G, and they are used when prolonged infusions are administered.

Large gauge (18 or 19) needles or catheters are used for administering blood or viscous liquids such as hyperalimentation fluid. For venipunctures on infants and children or for adults with small veins, a wing tip (butterfly) needle of suitable length may be used. On infants, a scalp vein butterfly needle may be preferable, Figure 10-1A.

Needleless IV devices that greatly reduce the risk of IV contamination via air, blood, or touch, and also reduce the risk of accidental needle-stick injuries are currently available, Figure 10-1B.

Infusion Sets

A variety of IV administration sets is available for use as primary setups for continuous infusion and secondary setups for intermittent infusion. All sets consist of intravenous tubing, some type of drip chamber, a roller clamp, and protective caps to maintain sterility.

The size of the opening into the drip chamber determines the size of the drop delivered by the infusion set. The most common sizes (called macrodrip) are calibrated to deliver 10, 15, or 20 drops per milliliter. Microdrip (minidrip) sets, calibrated to administer small and very precise amounts of fluid, deliver 60 drops per milliliter, Figure 10-2. The drop size, called the *drop factor,* is identified on the package. The drop factor refers to the

FIGURE 10-1A Needles and cannulas used for IVs

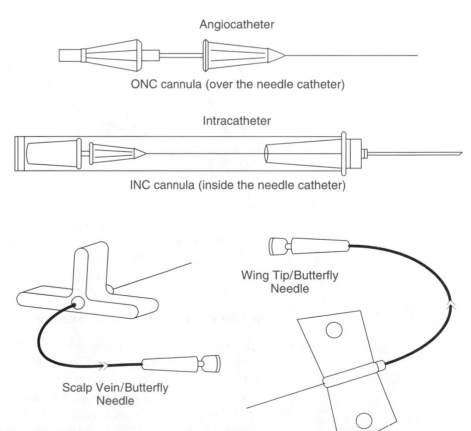

Angiocatheter

ONC cannula (over the needle catheter)

Intracatheter

INC cannula (inside the needle catheter)

Wing Tip/Butterfly Needle

Scalp Vein/Butterfly Needle

FIGURE 10-1B The PROTECTIV™ IV Catheter Safety System has built-in needlestick protection. As the user slides the catheter off the introducer needle, a protective guard glides over the contaminated needle before it is removed from the catheter hub. A reassuring "click" tells the user when the needle is locked safely inside the guard *(Courtesy Critikon, Inc.)*

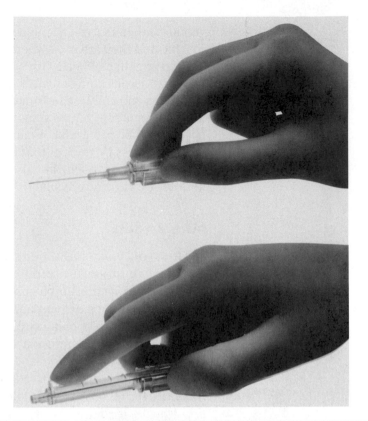

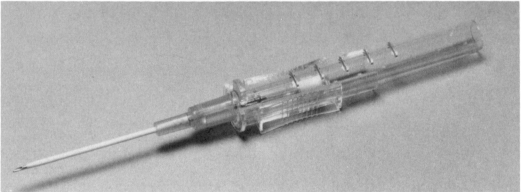

number of drops needed to deliver 1 mL of fluid, and always should be determined prior to calculating and/or adjusting the flow rate, Figure 10-3.

Infusion sets are adapted for use with vented or nonvented solution containers and may be used individually (primary line) or attached to each other (piggyback or secondary lines).

Intravenous Solution Containers

Intravenous solution containers are made of glass or plastic and come in a variety of sizes and shapes. Glass containers are vacuum sealed and have rubber stoppers with openings for the tubing, for venting, and/or for the addition of medications. Plastic containers have special ports for insertion of tubing and addition of medications. All containers are calibrated according to the amount of fluid contained and are labeled as to type of solution, instructions for use, and other pertinent information.

FIGURE 10-2   IV Drops

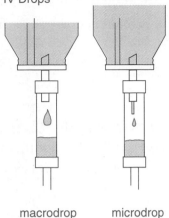

macrodrop   microdrop

FIGURE 10-3   *(Supplied by Baxter Healthcare Corporation, Deerfield, Illinois 50016 USA.* **Note: This product labeling is a sample and is subject to change at any time. Be sure to read the directions for use accompanying the product.***)*

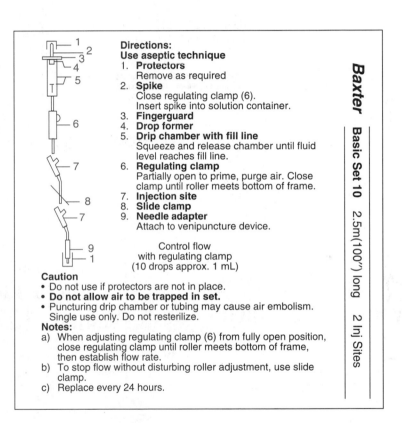

Directions:
Use aseptic technique
1. **Protectors**
   Remove as required
2. **Spike**
   Close regulating clamp (6).
   Insert spike into solution container.
3. **Fingerguard**
4. **Drop former**
5. **Drip chamber with fill line**
   Squeeze and release chamber until fluid level reaches fill line.
6. **Regulating clamp**
   Partially open to prime, purge air. Close clamp until roller meets bottom of frame.
7. **Injection site**
8. **Slide clamp**
9. **Needle adapter**
   Attach to venipuncture device.

Control flow
with regulating clamp
(10 drops approx. 1 mL)

Caution
• Do not use if protectors are not in place.
• **Do not allow air to be trapped in set.**
• Puncturing drip chamber or tubing may cause air embolism. Single use only. Do not resterilize.

Notes:
a) When adjusting regulating clamp (6) from fully open position, close regulating clamp until roller meets bottom of frame, then establish flow rate.
b) To stop flow without disturbing roller adjustment, use slide clamp.
c) Replace every 24 hours.

Baxter

Basic Set 10   2.5m(100") long   2 Inj Sites

Intravenous Solutions

Commonly used IV solutions and their abbreviations are:

Solution	*Abbreviation*
Water	W
Saline	S
Normal Saline	NS
Dextrose	D
Ringers Lactate	RL
Lactated Ringers	LR

Reading Labels:
Drop Factor

From Figure 10-4, answer the following questions:

1. What is the calibration in drops per milliliter (drop factor) for each of the infusion sets?

   a. _____

   b. _____

   c. _____

2. Which is/are macrodrip set(s)? _____

3. Which is/are microdrip (minidrip) set(s)? _____

(**Note:** See Appendix G for answer key.)

10 drops approx. 1 mL
2.5 m (100″) long

Caution: Federal (USA) law restricts this device
to sale by or on order of a physician.

2C5425 s

Baxter

Basic Set
10

a.

Nitroglycerin   No. 1772
Primary I.V. Set-SL
Vented, 107 Inch

ⓐ   15
                              DROPS/mL

b.

Nitroglycerin MICRODRIP®   No. 9252
IV Micro Pump Set-SL
Vented, 107 Inch

ⓐ   60
                           DROPS/mL
                           TYPE A

c.

FIGURE 10-4   *(Part a supplied by Baxter Healthcare Corporation, Deerfield Illinois 60015 USA.* **Note: This product labeling is a sample and is subject to change at any time. Be sure to read the directions for use accompanying the product.** *Parts b and c courtesy of Abbot Laboratories.)*

Reading IV Labels

Refer to Figure 10-5

1. What is the total amount of solution in the container? _____

2. What percentage of the solution is dextrose? _____ (this IV solution would be abbreviated D5W)

3. What is the name of the manufacturer? _____

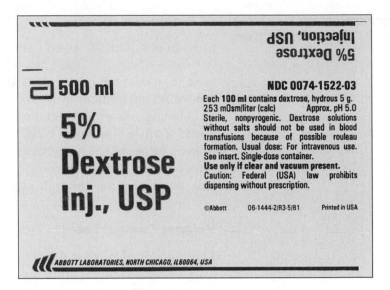

5% Dextrose
Injection, USP

NDC 0074-1522-03

Each **100 ml** contains dextrose, hydrous 5 g.
253 mOsm/liter (calc)   Approx. pH 5.0
Sterile, nonpyrogenic. Dextrose solutions
without salts should not be used in blood
transfusions because of possible rouleau
formation. Usual dose: For intravenous use.
See insert. Single-dose container.
Use only if clear and vacuum present.
Caution: Federal (USA) law prohibits
dispensing without prescription.

©Abbott   06-1444-2/R3-5/81   Printed in USA

Ⓐ 500 ml

5%

Dextrose

Inj., USP

ABBOTT LABORATORIES, NORTH CHICAGO, IL60064, USA

Refer to Figure 10-6

1. What is the total amount of solution in the container? _____

2. What percentage of the solution is Sodium Chloride?* _____
    *This percentage solution is also called Normal Saline and orders may
    be written using the abbreviation NS.

250 ml
0.9% Sodium Chloride
Inj., USP

Refer to Figure 10-7

1. What is the total amount of solution in the container? _____

2. What percentage of the solution is dextrose? _____ (this IV solu-
    tion would be abbreviated D5LR)

3. What other chemical ingredients does the solution contain? _____

(**Note:** See Appendix G for answer key.)

1000 ml
5% DEXTROSE AND LACTATED RINGERS
INJECTION, USP
Each 100 ml contains 600 mg
Sodium Chloride USP, 310 mg
Sodium Lactate, 30 mg Potassium
Chloride USP, 20 mg Calcium
Chloride USP

Intermittent IV Drug Administration

IV Piggyback (IVPB)

Medications often are given intravenously by adding a secondary infusion line to an existing IV line. This is called the piggyback method and often is used to administer medications that are ordered at regularly scheduled times (i.e., intermittent drug administration) (e.g., q 6 hr).

Medications administered via piggyback usually are diluted in 50–100 mL of solution. They may be infused simultaneously or alternately with a primary infusion. The piggyback set includes a small IV bottle or bag, a drip chamber, short tubing, and a needle (usually 20 gauge, 1″) that is inserted into the primary line through a special port, Figure 10-8.

Volume Control Set

This is a special infusion set designed to administer small amounts of fluid over a specified time period, usually 30–60 minutes. It consists of a small fluid chamber, drip chamber, and tubing, and can be used as either a primary or secondary infusion line, Figure 10-9. The fluid chamber holds 100

FIGURE 10-8
IV piggyback

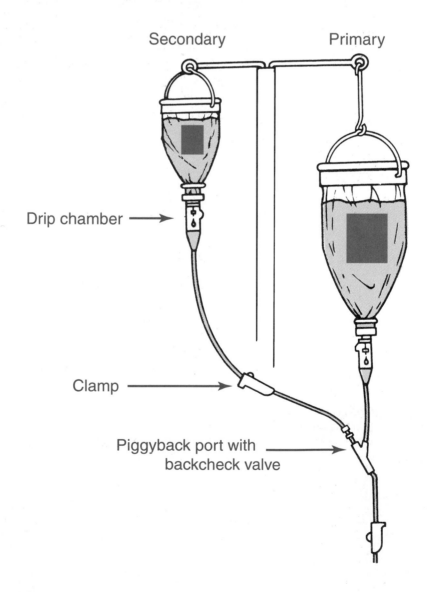

Secondary   Primary

Drip chamber →

Clamp →

Piggyback port with backcheck valve →

FIGURE 10-9   IV volume
control set

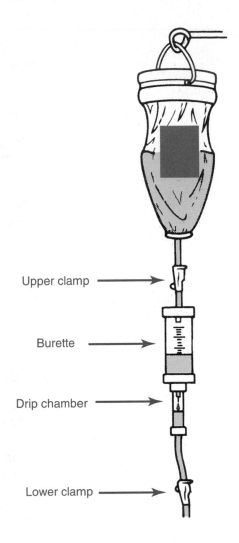

Upper clamp ⟶

Burette ⟶

Drip chamber ⟶

Lower clamp ⟶

mL or more, to which medications can be added through a medication port. The drip chamber is calibrated at 60 gtt/mL (micro- or minidrip) and the IV flow rate is regulated by adjusting the clamp below this chamber. These sets often are referred to by their brand names such as *Buretrol, Volutrol,* and *Metriset.*

Saline Lock

The saline lock, also called saline well, is a device that serves as an intermittent IV line. It may be used for administration of regularly scheduled IV medications for patients who do not also require parenteral fluids, thus eliminating the need for a continuous IV. Alternatively, a saline lock may be inserted for the purpose of administering IV medications that are incompatible with solutions or drugs concurrently being given IV.

The device consists of an IV needle or catheter attached to a short plastic tube that terminates in a rubber seal, Figure 10-10. Medication is injected or infused through the seal at the designated times. Because the needle or catheter remains in the vein, it must be flushed periodically with saline to prevent clot formation and to maintain patency. In some

FIGURE 10-10 Saline lock

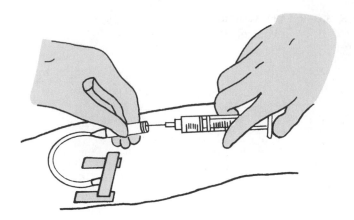

instances, depending on hospital policy, diluted heparin is injected following the saline flush. (The saline lock sometimes is referred to as the heparin lock.)

Central Venous Catheter

Medications can be infused through a catheter that is inserted into a major vein and usually advanced from this vein into the superior vena cava. If the catheter also is to be used for measuring central venous pressure, it is directed through the vena cava into the right atrium. Because the catheter is left in place, it can be used for a continuous or intermittent infusion line. Veins most commonly used for central venous lines are the subclavian and the external jugular, although the brachial and femoral veins are alternative routes.

A very useful modification of the central venous catheter is a multilumen catheter that permits a variety of treatment and monitoring procedures to be performed via a single venipuncture site.

One such device is pictured in Figure 10-11. This catheter, which contains three lumens, can be used in place of multiple central and peripheral lines for patients who require a multiplicity of intravenous therapy and monitoring, often several procedures simultaneously. This versatile central venous catheter provides routes for fluid administration, TPN (total parenteral nutrition), blood sampling, central venous pressure monitoring, and medication administration, including simultaneous infusion of incompatible drugs.

The multilumen catheter must be flushed periodically with saline to maintain patency of lumens that are used intermittently. The procedure is similar to that used with the saline lock. A lumen that is being used for a continuous IV infusion does not need to be flushed.

Electronic Infusion Regulators

Electronic infusion regulators are electronic pumps and controllers that help provide accuracy and safety in administration of IV therapy. Controllers automatically regulate the drop rate of infusions where the force of gravity provides the needed pressure to maintain fluid flow, Figure 10-12.

FIGURE 10-11
Multilumen central venous
catheter for CVP monitoring
and/or multiple infusions at one
puncture site *(Courtesy of Arrow
International, Inc.)*

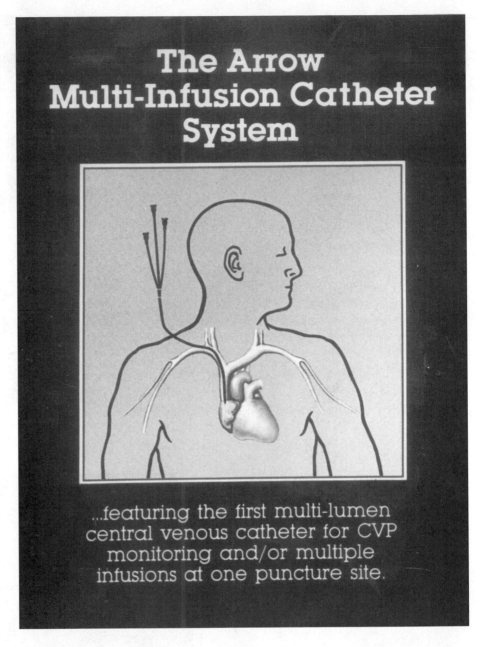

The Arrow Multi-Infusion Catheter System

...featuring the first multi-lumen central venous catheter for CVP monitoring and/or multiple infusions at one puncture site.

Pumps fall into two categories, the IV regulator pump and the syringe pump. The IV regulator pump maintains fluid flow by means of positive pressure, which can be varied or adjusted as needed, Figure 10-13. The syringe pump, also called a mini-infuser, is used when a small amount of medication (e.g., up to 60 mL) is administered. The medication is infused from a syringe that is inserted into the apparatus, Figure 10-14.

Pumps and controllers have a variety of mechanisms for automatically regulating drop rate and/or fluid volume and for providing warning alarms when there is a problem with the infusion or equipment.

If electronic (automatic) devices are not in use, the nurse manually sets and/or adjusts the flow rate to the desired gtt/min by use of a roller-clamp on the IV tubing.

FIGURE 10-12
Volumetric controller *(Courtesy IVAC Corporation)*

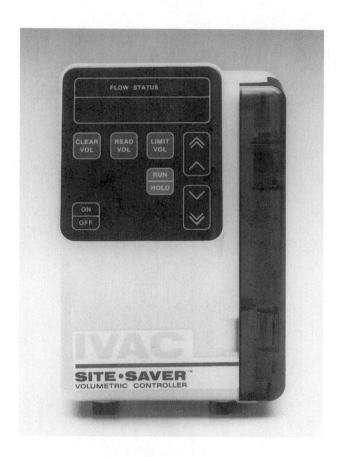

FIGURE 10-13 Variable pressure pump *(Courtesy IVAC Corporation)*

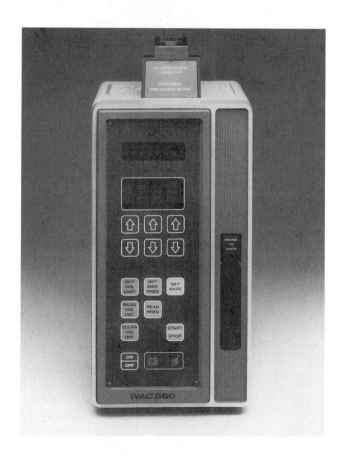

FIGURE 10-14   Harvard mini infuser *(Courtesy Bard® Med Systems Division.*

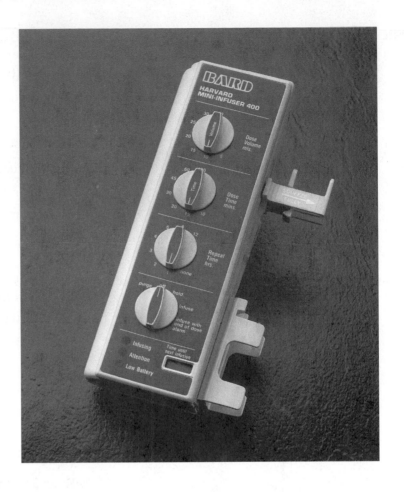

Calculation of Intravenous Flow Rates, Infusion Times, Infusion Rate, and Bolus Using Dimensional Analysis

Once the infusion is started, the nurse is responsible for regulating the flow rate (i.e., the number of drops per minute required to infuse the IV within the time period or infusion rate specified).

In calculating the flow rate for *drops per minute,* one minute becomes the labeled value that must be converted to an equivalent value: number of drops. *One minute,* therefore, is the starting factor and *drops* is the answer unit and these, as in all dimensional analysis conversions, form an equivalent relationship.

It is essential in calculating flow rate to know the drop factor. This refers to the size of the drop delivered by the particular infusion set being used: the number of drops required to make 1 mL (cc). The drop factor always will be stated in practice problems requiring calculation of drops per minute.

Rounding Off

The rate of flow should be rounded to the nearest whole number.

1. 31.6 gtt/min; adjust to 32 gtt/min
2. 42.3 gtt/min; adjust to 42 gtt/min
3. 56.8 mL/hr; adjust to 57 mL/hr
4. 120.4 mL/hr; adjust to 120 mL/hr

Calculation of IV Flow Rate When Total Infusion Time Is Specified

EXAMPLE

Order: 1000 mL of D5W (5% Dextrose in water) IV to infuse over a period of 5 hr

Drop Factor: 10 gtt/mL

Starting Factor	Answer Unit
1 min	gtt

Equivalents: 1000 mL = 5 hr, 10 gtt = 1 mL, 60 min = 1 hr

Conversion Equation:

$$1 \, \text{min} \times \frac{1 \, \text{hr}}{60 \, \text{min}} \times \frac{1000 \, \text{mL}}{5 \, \text{hr}} \times \frac{10 \, \text{gtt}}{1 \, \text{mL}} = 33.3 = 33 \, \text{gtt}$$

Flow Rate: 33 gtt/min

Calculation of IV Flow Rate When an Infusion Rate Is Specified

EXAMPLES

Order: 1500 mL of Sodium Chloride 0.9% (0.9% Sodium Chloride Solution) to infuse at a rate of 90 mL/hr

Drop Factor: 20 gtt/mL

Starting Factor	Answer Unit
1 min	gtt

Equivalents: 90 mL = 1 hr, 20 gtt = 1 mL, 60 min = 1 hr

Conversion Equation:

$$1 \, \text{min} \times \frac{1 \, \text{hr}}{60 \, \text{min}} \times \frac{90 \, \text{mL}}{1 \, \text{hr}} \times \frac{20 \, \text{gtt}}{1 \, \text{mL}} = 30 \, \text{gtt}$$

Flow Rate: 33 gtt/min

EXAMPLE

Order: 1000 mL of 5% D ½ NSS (5% Dextrose in ½ Normal Saline Solution) to infuse at a rate of 100 mL/hr

Drop Factor: 60 gtt/mL

Starting Factor	Answer Unit
1 min	gtt

Equivalents: 100 mL = 1 hr, 60 gtt = 1 mL, 60 min = 1 hr

Conversion Equation:

$$1 \, \text{min} \times \frac{1 \, \text{hr}}{60 \, \text{min}} \times \frac{100 \, \text{mL}}{1 \, \text{hr}} \times \frac{60 \, \text{gtt}}{1 \, \text{mL}} = 100 \, \text{gtt}$$

*Flow rate: 100 gtt/min

***Note:** When using any infusion set having a drop factor of 60 gtt/mL (sometimes written as: drop factor microdrip), the flow rate per minute *always* will be the same as the number of mL per hour. For example:

Order: 50 mL/hr; flow rate: 50 gtt/min

Order: 70 mL/hr; flow rate: 70 gtt/min

Therefore, the flow rate calculation can be omitted for this type of order.

EXAMPLE   **Order:** 500 mL D5W IV KVO

The abbreviation KVO stands for Keep Vein Open (or TKO = To Keep Open). This means that the IV is to run at a very slow rate simply to have an infusion route available for emergency use or intermittent administration of drugs. A microdrip infusion set usually is used. A typical flow rate, which may vary according to hospital policy, is 10–20 mL/hr.

It can be seen from the box above that no calculation is necessary for a KVO order, because the flow rate will be the same as the stated mL/hr; in the case, 10–20 gtt/min.

PRACTICE
Calculation of IV Flow Rate When Total Infusion Time Is Specified

1. **Order:** 1500 mL of D5W IV to infuse in 8 hr
   Drop Factor: 10 gtt/mL

2. **Order:** 1000 mL NS to infuse in 10 hr
   Drop Factor: 15 gtt/mL

3. **Order:** 800 mL 5% glucose in water in 4 hr
   Drop Factor: 15 gtt/mL

4. **Order:** 700 mL D5W IV in 5 hr
   Drop Factor: 10 gtt/mL

5. **Order:** 2500 mL 5% Dextrose in 0.45 NS IV in 24 hr
   Drop Factor: 20 gtt/mL

6. **Order:** 1250 mL d 2.5 W IV in 6 hr
Drop Factor: 15 gtt/mL

7. **Order:** 500 mL Sodium Chloride 0.9% IV in 3 hr
Drop Factor: 10 gtt/mL

8. **Order:** 100 mL Ringers IV in 4 hr
Drop Factor: 15 gtt/mL

9. **Order:** 300 mL D5W IV in 3 hr
Drop Factor: 60 gtt/mL

10. **Order:** 50 cc Serum Albumin IV to infuse in 1 hr
Drop Factor: 15 gtt/mL

PRACTICE
Calculation of IV Flow Rate When an Infusion Rate Is Specified

11. **Order:** 1000 mL Ringers IV to infuse at a rate of 125 mL/hr
Drop Factor: 15 gtt/mL
What should the flow rate be per minute?

12. **Order:** 1000 mL D5W IV to infuse at a rate of 100 mL/hr
Drop Factor: 10 gtt/mL
What should the flow rate be per minute?

13. **Order:** 1500 mL Sodium Chloride 0.9% IV to infuse at a rate of 150 mL/hr
Drop Factor: 15 gtt/mL
What should the flow rate be per minute?

14. **Order:** 2000 mL of D2.5W IV to infuse at a rate of 125 mL/hr
Drop Factor: 10 gtt/mL
What should the flow rate be per minute?

15. **Order:** 500 mL Isolyte M IV to infuse at a rate of 125 mL/hr
Drop Factor: 60 gtt/mL
What should the flow rate be per minute?

16. **Order:** Hyperalimentation (TPN) 1000 mL D20W IV to infuse at a rate of 80 mL/hr
Drop Factor: 15 gtt/mL
What should the flow rate be per minute?

17. **Order:** Hyperalimentation (TPN) 1000 mL Aminosyn 3.5% IV to infuse at a rate of 40 mL/hr
Drop Factor: 20 gtt/mL
What should the flow rate be per minute?

(**Note:** See Appendix G for answer key.)

Calculation of Flow Rate (gtt/min) When IV Contains Medication

The IV flow rate is calculated the same whether or not medication has been added to the IV container. If medication is to be added, however, the additional numbers in the order may cause confusion in determining the conversion factors. It is, therefore, essential to carefully inspect the information given and select the correct equivalents for the conversion equation.

EXAMPLE

Order: Ampicillin 500 mg in 50 mL of Sodium Chloride 0.9% to infuse in 1 hr.

Drop Factor: 60 gtt/mL

Starting Factor	Answer Unit
1 min	gtt

Equivalents: 50 mL = 1 hr, 60 gtt = 1 mL, 60 min = 1 hr

Conversion Equation:

$$1 \text{ min} \times \frac{1 \text{ hr}}{60 \text{ min}} \times \frac{50 \text{ mL}}{1 \text{ hr}} \times \frac{60 \text{ gtt}}{1 \text{ mL}} = 50 \text{ gtt}$$

Flow Rate: 50 gtt/min

(**Note:** The medication (Ampicillin 500 mg) that is added to the total amount of IV solution (50 mL) and the 0.9% NaCl are not pertinent to the computation of the flow rate and are not included in the conversion equation.)

PRACTICE
Calculation of Flow Rate When IV Contains Medication

1. **Order:** 1000 mL D5NS with KCl 40 mEq IV to infuse in 4 hr
   Drop Factor: 15 gtt/mL

2. **Order:** 250 mL D5W with Aminophylline 0.5 g IV to infuse in 2 hr
   Drop Factor: 60 gtt/mL

3. **Order:** Geopen (carbenicillin disodium) 2 g in 50 mL Sodium Chloride 0.9% to infuse in 30 min
   Drop Factor: 15 gtt/mL

4. **Order:** Erythromycin 500 mg in 100 mL D5W to infuse in 20 min
   Drop Factor: 10 gtt/mL

5. **Order:** Cleocin (clindamycin) 600 mg in 100 mL D5W to infuse in 60 min
   Drop Factor: 20 gtt/mL

(**Note:** See Appendix G for answer key.)

Calculation of IV Flow Rate When an Infusion Pump Is Used

Intravenous (infusion) pumps are useful, because they maintain a more accurate flow rate than is possible with the standard IV (gravity) administration set. The most commonly used pumps are volumetric and nonvolumetric.

Nonvolumetric pumps are designed to administer a certain number of drops per minute. The flow rate is determined in gtt/min and the pump is set to deliver this amount. Nonvolumetric pumps have been replaced by volumetric systems for the most part.

Volumetric pumps are designed to administer fluid in milliliters per hour. The flow rate is determined in mL/hr and the corresponding gtt/min rate is determined from a conversion chart that usually is printed on the infusion apparatus.

EXAMPLE **Order:** 500 mL D5½NS IV to infuse at a 10 hr rate (i.e., over a period of 10 hr). Use an infusion pump.

How many mL/hr should be administered?

Starting Factor	Answer Unit
1 hr	mL

Equivalents: 500 mL = 10 hr

Conversion Equation: $1 \, \cancel{hr} \times \dfrac{500 \text{ mL}}{10 \, \cancel{hr}} = 50 \text{ mL}$

The number of *drops per minute* required to deliver this amount of *solution per hour* depends on the drop factor of the tubing being used (e.g., 10-15-20-60 gtt/mL). In this case, because an infusion pump is being used, the drops per minute would be determined by consulting the operating manual or a conversion chart on the pump, Table 10-1.

Find the drops/min setting for the above flow rate (50 mL/hr). The infusion set has a tubing drop factor of 20 gtt/mL.

Answer: The pump would be set to deliver 17 gtt/min.

TABLE 10-1   Conversion between mL/hr and gtt/min

Desired Rate mL/hr	gtt/min Setting			
	Tubing Drop Factor			
	10	15	20	60
10	2	3	3	10
20	3	5	7	20
30	5	8	10	30
40	7	10	13	40
50	8	13	17	50
60	10	15	20	60

PRACTICE
Calculation of the Number of mL/hr That Will Infuse

1. **Order:** 1000 mL 5% D/NS IV to infuse at an 8 hr rate

2. **Order:** 500 mL Lactated Ringers IV to infuse at a 6 hr rate

3. **Order:** 1500 mL 2.5% D 0.45 NaCl IV to infuse at a 12 hr rate

4. **Order:** 250 mL D 2.5/W IV to infuse at a 2 hr rate

5. **Order:** 2500 mL NS IV to infuse at a 24 hr rate

6. **Order:** Hyperalimentation (TPN) 2000 mL Liposyn II 20% IV to infuse in 24 hr

7. **Order:** Hyperalimentation (TPN) 3000 mL Aminosyn 8.5% IV to infuse in 24 hr

___

(**Note:** See Appendix G for answer key.)

Calculation of Infusion Time

Dimensional Analysis can be used to calculate the anticipated length of time required for an infusion to be completed. (**Note:** When doing these problems, carry answers to hundredths and round to tenths. Convert to hr or min.)

EXAMPLE   **Order:** 1500 mL D2.5W IV
Drop Factor: 15 gtt/mL
Flow Rate: 40 gtt/min
How many hours will it take for the IV to infuse?

In this problem, the value sought is the length of time required to infuse a certain amount. The unit of time, therefore, becomes the answer unit. The quantity that will be converted to a unit of time (1500 mL) becomes the starting factor. The conversion equation is set up and solved in the usual manner.

Starting Factor Answer Unit
1500 mL   hours

Equivalents: 15 gtt = 1 mL, 40 gtt = 1 min, 60 min = 1 hr

Conversion Equation:

$$1500 \text{ mL} \times \frac{15 \text{ gtt}}{1 \text{ mL}} \times \frac{1 \text{ min}}{40 \text{ gtt}} \times \frac{1 \text{ hr}}{60 \text{ min}} = 9.4$$

$$= 9 \text{ hr } 24 \text{ min*}$$

*Convert the decimal to minutes by multiplying by 60.

PRACTICE
Calculation of Infusion Time

1. **Order:** 1500 mL Lactated Ringers IV
   Drop Factor: 10 gtt/mL
   Flow Rate: 20 gtt/min
   How long should it take the IV to infuse?

2. **Order:** 750 mL D10W IV
   Drop Factor: 15 gtt/mL
   Flow Rate: 21 gtt/min
   How long should it take the IV to infuse?

3. **Order:** 500 mL of Sodium Chloride 0.9% IV
   Drop Factor: 60 gtt/mL
   Flow Rate: 125 gtt/min
   How long should it take the IV to infuse?

4. **Order:** 2000 mL D5W
   Drop Factor: 15 gtt/mL
   Flow Rate: 34 gtt/min
   How long should it take the IV to infuse?

5. **Order:** 1000 mL D2.5NS IV
   Drop Factor: 10 gtt/mL
   Flow Rate: 23 gtt/min
   How long should it take the IV to infuse?

(**Note:** See Appendix G for answer key.)

Adding Medications to Intravenous Fluids

Intravenous medications can be administered in several ways. They may be added directly to a traditional IV set up, called a primary line, for continuous drip. For intermittent doses (e.g., every 8 or 12 hours), medications may be added to a second line that is then connected to the primary line, or they may be infused through a central venous line. Medications also can be injected directly into a vein (IV bolus) using a syringe and needle; through a primary line via the flashball or a Y-port; or through a saline lock. The medication order should state clearly the desired IV route of administration.

If two or more medications are added to the same IV, it is essential that the substances be compatible. The person mixing and adding substances to an IV has responsibility for ascertaining compatibility. Information about drug compatibility is obtained from the pharmacist, a drug reference book, the manufacturer's product insert, or a drug incompatibility chart.

Whenever a substance is added to an IV, the container must be labeled with the name, dosage, date, and time added.

Medications that are dispensed in liquid form may be added to the IV container through a medication port for infusion or through the tubing or saline lock for injection. Medications that are dispensed as dry powders or crystals must be reconstituted just prior to infusion or injection. Instructions for reconstitution are printed in the package insert or on the medication label. Reconstitution and mixing of intravenous medications usually is done by a registered pharmacist in a controlled area (e.g., under laminar air flow hood) in the pharmacy. Nurses may add medication to existing infusions, but rarely reconstitute.

Remember that only solvents designated in the directions should be used for reconstitution, because these have been determined to be compatible with this particular drug. In addition, when reconstituted drugs are added to IV solutions, it is likewise essential that drug and solution are compatible.

Depending on the amount (volume) of drug that is added to an IV, the total amount of solution to be administered may need to be adjusted in writing the conversion equation for determining flow rate. Several methods may be used. The practitioner may choose the method most appropriate to the situation, depending on hospital policy which may require or omit application of the 5% rule (a and b below).

a. If the amount (volume) of drug to be added is 5% or more of the total amount ordered to be administered, add the two amounts together in the conversion equation.

b. If the amount (volume) of drug to be added is less than 5% of the total amount ordered to be administered, this amount usually is considered negligible and it is not necessary to add the two amounts together in the conversion equation.

c. Remove from the IV container an amount of solution sufficient to reconstitute a powdered drug, then return the reconstituted solution to the container, thus not significantly changing the ordered quantity to be administered.

d. Remove from the IV container and discard an amount of solution equal to that which will be replaced by the ordered amount (volume) of drug. This approach is especially desirable in situations where fluid intake is strictly limited and/or measured.

Adding Drugs to IVs and Calculating Flow Rate in gtt/min

EXAMPLE

Order: Vibramycin 75 mg in 1000 mL Normosol-M in D5W IV to run in 24 hr

Label: Vibramycin (doxycycline hyclate) 100 mg (Figure 10-15)

Directions for reconstitution: Add 10 mL sterile water for injection to yield a concentration of 10 mg/mL.

a. How much of the reconstituted solution must be added to the IV bottle to provide the ordered dose of Vibramycin 75 mg?

Equivalent: 10 mg = 1 mL

Conversion Equation: $75 \text{ mg} \times \dfrac{1 \text{ mL}}{10 \text{ mg}} = 7.5 \text{ mL}$

Add Vibramycin 7.5 mL to 1000 mL Normosol-M in D5W.

FIGURE 10-15

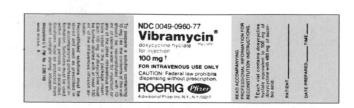

b. What should the flow rate be for this IV order? (Use 5% rule.)

Drop Factor: 15 gtt/mL

Equivalents: 1000 mL = 24 hr, 60 min = 1 hr, 15 gtt = 1 mL

Conversion Equation:

$$1\ \cancel{min} \times \frac{1\ \cancel{hr}}{60\ \cancel{min}} \times \frac{1000\ \cancel{mL}}{24\ \cancel{hr}} \times \frac{15\ gtt}{1\ \cancel{mL}} = 10.4$$
$$= 10\ gtt$$

Note: Because the 7.5 mL of reconstituted drug is less than 5% of the total volume (1000 mL) ordered to be administered, it is not necessary to add these amounts together in the conversion equation.

EXAMPLE

Order: Ticar 3 g in 100 mL Lactated Ringers IV to run in 2 hr

Label: Ticar (ticarcillin disodium) 3 g

Directions for reconstituting: Add 12 mL sterile water for injection to yield a concentration of 200 mg/mL.

a. How much of the reconstituted solution must be added to the IV bottle to provide the ordered dose of Ticar 3 g?

Equivalents: 1 g = 1000 mg   200 mg = 1 mL

Conversion Equation:

$$3\ \cancel{g} \times \frac{1000\ \cancel{mg}}{1\ \cancel{g}} \times \frac{1\ mL}{200\ \cancel{mg}} = 15\ mL$$

Add Ticar 15 mL to 100 mL Lactated Ringers Solution

b. What should the flow rate be for this IV order? (Use 5% rule.)

Drop Factor: 60 gtt/mL

Equivalents: 1 hr = 60 min   115 mL = 2 hr
60 gtt = 1 mL

Conversion Equation:

$$1\ \cancel{min} \times \frac{1\ \cancel{hr}}{60\ \cancel{min}} \times \frac{115\ \cancel{mL}}{2\ \cancel{hr}} \times \frac{60\ gtt}{1\ \cancel{mL}} = 57.5 = 58\ gtt$$

Note: Because the 15 mL of reconstituted drug is greater than 5% of the total volume (100 mL) ordered to be administered, it is necessary to add these amounts together in the conversion equation.

PRACTICE
Adding Drugs to IVs and Calculating Flow Rate in gtt/min

FIGURE 10-16

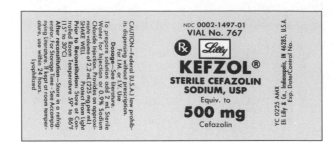

1. **Order:** Kefzol 350 mg in 100 mL 5% D/LR IV to run in 60 min.
   Label: Figure 10-16. What is the generic name? _____
   Drop Factor: 15 gtt/mL

   a. How much diluent must be added to the vial to reconstitute the drug for intravenous use?

   b. How much of the resulting solution must be added to the IV bottle to provide the ordered dose of Kefzol 350 mg?

   c. What should the flow rate be for this IV order? (Use 5% rule.)

FIGURE 10-17

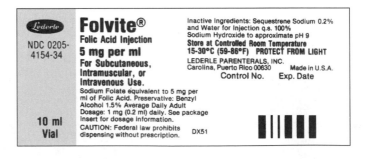

2. **Order:** Folic Acid 12 mg in 500 mL D5W in 4 hours
   Label: Figure 10-17
   Drop Factor: 60 gtt/mL

a. How many mL of Folvite must be added to the IV bottle to provide the ordered dose?

b. What should the flow rate be for this IV order? (Use 5% rule.)

FIGURE 10-18

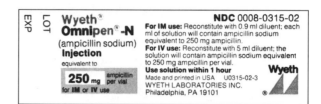

3. **Order:** Ampicillin Sodium 150 mg in 1000 mL M/6 Sodium Lactate IV to infuse at a rate of 150 mL/hr
Label: Figure 10-18. What is the trade name? _____
Drop Factor: 15 gtt/mL

a. How many mL of Ampicillin Sodium must be added to the IV bottle to provide the total ordered dose?

b. What should the flow rate be to administer the ordered number of mL/hr?

FIGURE 10-19

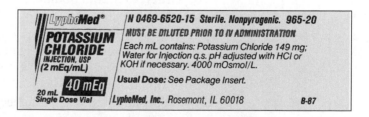

4. **Order:** Potassium Chloride (KCl) 30 mEq in 1000 mL D5NS IV in 6 hr
Label: Potassium Chloride (KCl) injection 40 mEq in 20 mL vial, Figure 10-19

(**Note:** This medication is already in solution; therefore, reconstitution is not necessary.)

Drop Factor: 10 gtt/mL

a. How many mL of this medication must be added to the IV bottle to provide the ordered dose of KCl 30 mEq?

b. What should the flow rate be for this IV order? (Use 5% rule.)

5. **Order:** Tetracycline 150 mg in 100 mL Sodium Chloride 0.9% to infuse in 40 min via Volutrol
Label: Tetracycline 250 mg
Directions: Dilute with 5 mL sterile water for injection and add to ordered IV solution.
Drop Factor: 60 gtt/mL

a. How many mL of the reconstituted solution should be added to the IV solution?

b. What should the flow rate be for this IV order? (Use 5% rule.)

6. **Order:** Cefoxitin Sodium 2 g IV in 100 mL Lactated Ringers Solution to infuse in 60 min
Label: Cefoxitin Sodium 2 g
Directions: Reconstitute with 20 mL sterile water for injection to yield 2 g/21 mL.
Drop factor: 60 gtt/mL
What should the flow rate be? (Use 5% rule.)

7. **Order:** Ampicillin Sodium 250 mg IVPB in 100 mL D5W to infuse in 60 min
   Label: Ampicillin Sodium 1 g
   Directions: Reconstitute with 3.5 mL sterile water for injection to yield 1 g/4 mL.
   Drop Factor: 10 gtt/mL

   a. How many mL of the reconstituted solutions should be added to the IV solution?

   b. What should the flow rate be? (Use 5% rule.)

8. **Order:** Coly-Mycin M 100 mg in 500 mL D5W to infuse at 5 mg/hr
   Label: Coly-Mycin M (colistimethate sodium) 150 mg
   Directions: Reconstitute with 2 mL sterile water for injection to yield 75 mg/mL and add to IV solution.
   Drop factor: 60 gtt/mL

   a. How many mL of reconstituted solution should be added to the IV solution?

   b. What should the flow rate be? (Use 5% rule.)

9. **Order:** Mithracin 1534 mcg in 1000 mL D5W to infuse in 6 hr
   Label: Mithracin (plicamycin) 2.5 mg
   Directions: Reconstitute with 4.9 mL of sterile water for injection to yield 0.5 mg/mL and add to IV solution.
   Drop Factor: 60 gtt/mL

   a. How many mL of reconstituted Mithracin should be added to the ordered IV solution?

   b. What should the flow rate be? (Use 5% rule.)

10. **Order:** Penicillin G Potassium 5 million units in 100 mL D5W IV to infuse over 1 hr
    Label: Penicillin G Potassium 20,000,000 U dry powder
    Directions: Reconstitute with 31.6 mL sterile water for injection to yield concentration of 500,000 U/mL.
    Drop Factor: 15 gtt/mL

    a. How many mL of the reconstituted Penicillin G should be added to the 100 mL D5W?

    b. What should the flow rate be? (Omit 5% rule.)

(**Note:** See Appendix G for answer key.)

Critical Care
IV Calculations

Adding Drugs to IVs and Calculating the Drug Infusion Rate

The physician may order the IV medication to be infused at the rate of a specified concentration (amount) of drug per unit of time. We call this the drug infusion rate.

The drug infusion rate can be calculated in terms of either:

a. *volume of solution* per unit of time (e.g., mL/hr or mL/min)

   OR

b. *concentration of drug* per unit of time (e.g., mg, mcg, U/hr or min).

EXAMPLE   A drug infusion rate of 2.5 U/hr means that:

a. the IV flow rate (volume/unit of time) that will infuse 2.5 U of the drug per hour must be determined

   OR

b. the concentration of drug contained in a specified amount of solution per hour must be determined.

Because these are usually potent drugs that require the most accurate method of infusion, they are administered using a microdrip infusion set and volumetric infusion pump. Because the pump mL/hr rate corresponds to the microdrip/min rate, the IV flow rate can be calculated in mL/hr and the corresponding gtt/min setting selected (see Table 10-1). This will automatically infuse the correct amount per hour or per minute.

EXAMPLE   **Order:** Heparin 20,000 U in 500 mL Sodium Chloride 0.9% IV to infuse at 1200 U/hr. Use an infusion pump.

How many mL/hr should be administered?

Starting Factor   Answer Unit
       1 hr   mL

Equivalents: 1200 U = 1 hr   20,000 U = 500 mL
Conversion Equation:

$$1\ \cancel{hr} \times \frac{1200\ \cancel{U}}{1\ \cancel{hr}} \times \frac{500\ mL}{20,000\ \cancel{U}} = 30\ mL$$

Flow Rate: 30 mL/hr

Set the infusion pump at the gtt/min setting that corresponds to 30 mL/hr.

EXAMPLE   **Order:** Heparin 20,000 U in 500 mL Sodium Chloride 0.9% IV to infuse at 30 mL/hr.

How many Units will be infused per hour?

Starting Factor   Answer Unit
       1 hr   U

Equivalents: 30 mL = 1 hr   20,000 U = 500 mL

Conversion Equation:

$$1 \, \cancel{hr} \times \frac{30 \, \cancel{mL}}{1 \, \cancel{hr}} \times \frac{20,000 \, U}{500 \, \cancel{mL}} = 1200 \, U$$

EXAMPLE

Order: Aminophylline 280 mg in 350 mL D5W into central venous catheter. Infuse 250 mL in 75 min and the remainder at 20 mL/hr. Use an infusion pump.

Label: See Figure 10-20

1. How many mL of medication should be added to the IV bottle?

   Equivalents: 500 mg = 20 mL

   Conversion Equation:

   $$280 \, \cancel{mg} \times \frac{20 \, mL}{500 \, \cancel{mg}} = 11.2 \, mL$$

   Answer: Add Aminophylline 11.2 mL to 350 mL D5W.

2. How many mg would the patient receive per minute at the infusion rate of 250 mL/75 min?

   Equivalents: 250 mL = 75 min   350 mL = 280 mg

   Conversion Equation:

   $$1 \, \cancel{min} \times \frac{250 \, \cancel{mL}}{75 \, \cancel{min}} \times \frac{280 \, mg}{350 \, \cancel{mL}} = 2.7 \, mg$$

3. Determine the mL/hr to which the infusion pump should be set to infuse the first 250 mL of IV solution at the ordered rate.

   Equivalents: 60 min = 1 hr   250 mL = 75 min

   Conversion Equation:

   $$1 \, \cancel{hr} \times \frac{60 \, \cancel{min}}{1 \, \cancel{hr}} \times \frac{250 \, mL}{75 \, \cancel{min}} = 200 \, mL$$

   Answer: Regulate the infusion pump to deliver 200 mL/hr.

FIGURE 10-20

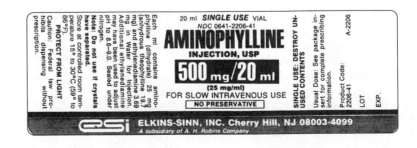

4. How long will it take to infuse the remaining solution at the ordered rate?

Equivalent: 20 mL = 1 hr

Conversion Equation:

$$100 \, \cancel{mL} \times \frac{1 \, hr}{20 \, \cancel{mL}} = 5 \, hr$$

PRACTICE
Calculation of the Volume of Solution or Concentration of Drug

1. **Order:** Pitocin 25 U in 1000 mL Sodium Chloride 0.9% IV to infuse at a drug infusion rate of 2.5 U/hr
   Label: Pitocin (oxytocin) 10 U/mL

   a. How many mL of Pitocin must be added to the IV bottle?

   b. How many mL/hr should be administered? (Use 5% rule.)

2. **Order:** Regular Insulin 100 U in 500 mL Sodium Chloride 0.9% to infuse at 5 U/hr via IV pump
   How many mL/hr should be administered?

3. **Order:** Morphine Sulfate 100 mg in 250 mL D5W to infuse at 3.2 mg/hr via IV pump
   How many mL/hr should be administered?

4. **Order:** Heparin 20,000 U in 1000 mL Sodium Chloride 0.9% to infuse at 1000 U/hr via IV pump
   How many mL/hr should be administered?

5. **Order:** Minocin (minocycline) 100 mg in 500 mL D5W to infuse at 20 mg/hr via IV pump
   How many mL/hr should be administered?

6. **Order:** Coly-Mycin-M 150 mg in 100 mL D5W to infuse in 60 minutes (via IV mini-bottle/saline lock)
   Label: Coly-Mycin-M (colestimethate sodium) 150 mg
   Directions: Reconstitute with 2 mL sterile water for injection to yield 75 mg/mL and add to ordered amount of IV solution.
   How many mL/hr should be administered?

7. **Order:** Cefizox 1 g in 50 mL Ringers Solution IV to infuse in 30 min via IV pump
   Label: Cefizox (ceftizoxime sodium) 1 g
   Directions: Reconstitute with 10 mL sterile water for injection to yield 1 g/10.7 mL.
   How many mL/hr should be administered via the IV pump? (Use 5% rule.)

8. **Order:** Pyopen 3 g in 100 mL D5W into central venous catheter to infuse in 90 min (use an infusion pump)
   Label: Pyopen (carbenicillin disodium) 5 g
   Directions: Reconstitute with 7 mL sterile water for injection to yield 500 mg/mL.

   a. How many mL of reconstituted solution should be added to the IV solution?

   b. How many mL/hr should be administered via the IV pump? (Omit 5% rule.)

9. **Order:** Cleocin 300 mg IV (Buretrol) in 50 mL D5W to infuse at dose rate of 30 mg/min (use an infusion pump)
   Label: Cleocin (clindamycin) 300 mg/2 mL
   Directions: Dilute in 50 mL of D5W and administer via volume control set.

a. Determine the mL/hr to which the infusion pump should be set.

b. At this rate, how many minutes will it take to infuse the ordered 50 mL?

10. **Order:** Aminophylline 500 mg in 500 mL D5W in 10 hr via IV pump
How many mg will infuse in 1 hr?

11. **Order:** Lidocaine 2 g in 500 mL D5W to infuse at 60 mL/hr via IV pump
How many mg will infuse in 1 min?

12. **Order:** Isuprel (isoproterenol HCl) 2 mg in 500 mL D5W to infuse at 45 mL/hr via IV pump
How many mcg will infuse in 1 min?

13. **Order:** KCl 10 mEq in 1000 mL D5½NS to infuse at 125 mL/hr via IV pump
How many mEq will infuse in 1 hr?

14. **Order:** Dopamine 400 mg in 250 mL D5W to infuse at 60 mL/hr via IV pump
How many mg will infuse in 1 hr?

15. **Order:** Aminophylline 250 mg in 250 mL D5W into central venous catheter. Infuse 200 mL in 45 minutes and the remainder at 17 mL/hr. Use an IV pump.
Label: Aminophylline 250 mg/10 mL

    a. How many mL of medication should be added to the IV bottle?

b. Determine the mL/hr to which the IV pump should be set to infuse the first 200 mL of solution at the ordered rate.

c. How long will it take to infuse the remaining solution at the ordered rate?

16. **Order:** Magnesium Sulfate 20 g in 1000 mL D5W IV via pump. Infuse 600 mL in 90 min and the remainder (400 mL) at 50 mL/hr
    Label: Magnesium Sulfate 5 g/10 mL

   a. How many mL should be added to the IV?

   b. How many g would the patient receive per minute at the infusion rate of 600 mL/90 min?

   c. Determine the mL/hr to which the IV pump should be set to infuse the first 600 mL of solution at the ordered rate.

   d. How long will it take to infuse the remaining solution at the ordered rate?

17. **Order:** Ritadrine Hydrochloride 150 mg in 500 mL Ringers IV (via IV pump) to infuse at 0.1 mg/min and increase by 0.05 mg/min every 10 min until uterine contractions cease
    Label: Ritadrine HCl 50 mg/5 mL

    a. How many mL of the medication should be added to the IV bottle?

    b. What is the concentration of the resulting solution per mL (i.e., mg of Ritadrine/mL)?

    c. How many mL/hr should be administered to infuse the initial dose of 0.1 mg/min? (Use 5% rule.)

    d. Ten minutes later, the flow rate should be increased to how many mL/hr to infuse the ordered dose (0.1 mg + 0.05 mg = 0.15 mg)? (Use 5% rule.)

    e. Ten minutes later, the flow rate should be increased to how many mL/hr to infuse the ordered dose (0.15 mg + 0.05 mg = 0.2 mg)? (Use 5% rule.)

(**Note:** See Appendix G for answer key.)

Calculating IV Dosage and Flow Rate Based on Body Weight

IV medications may be ordered according to a *specified amount* (e.g., mcg/kg of body weight) to be administered within a *specified unit* of time (e.g., per minute). The medication is added to a *specified volume* and type of IV solution. The total desired dose per minute must first be determined and then the infusion rate calculated that will administer the correct mL/hr or gtt/min. As a rule, a microdrip infusion set (60 gtt/mL) is used, along with an IV pump or controller.

EXAMPLE

Order: Infuse Nipride (nitroprusside sodium) 50 mg in 500 mL D5W at 3 mcg/kg/min

Weight: 215 lb

Drop Factor: 60 gtt/mL

1. How many mcg/min must be administered?

$$215 \text{ lb} \times \frac{1 \text{ kg}}{2.2 \text{ lb}} \times \frac{3 \text{ mcg/min}}{1 \text{ kg}} = 293.2 \text{ mcg/min}$$

2. How many mL/hr will provide the required dose?

$$1 \text{ hr} \times \frac{60 \text{ min}}{1 \text{ hr}} \times \frac{293.2 \text{ mcg}}{1 \text{ min}} \times \frac{1 \text{ mg}}{1000 \text{ mcg}} \times \frac{500 \text{ mL}}{50 \text{ mg}} = 175.9$$
$$= 176 \text{ mL/hr}$$

3. How many gtt/min will provide the required dose?

$$1 \text{ min} \times \frac{293.2 \text{ mcg}}{1 \text{ min}} \times \frac{1 \text{ mg}}{1000 \text{ mcg}} \times \frac{500 \text{ mL}}{50 \text{ mg}} \times \frac{60 \text{ gtt}}{1 \text{ mL}} = 175.9$$
$$= 176 \text{ gtt/min}$$

*OR

$$215 \text{ lb} \times \frac{1 \text{ kg}}{2.2 \text{ lb}} \times \frac{3 \text{ mcg}}{1 \text{ kg}} \times \frac{1 \text{ mg}}{1000 \text{ mcg}} \times \frac{500 \text{ mL}}{50 \text{ mg}} \times \frac{60 \text{ gtt}}{1 \text{ mL}} = 175.9$$
$$= 176 \text{ gtt/min}$$

4. How many mcg/gtt will be administered?

$$1 \text{ gtt} \times \frac{1 \text{ min}}{176 \text{ gtt}} \times \frac{293.2 \text{ mcg}}{1 \text{ min}} = 1.7 \text{ mcg/gtt}$$

***Note:** When calculating gtt/min, the step of calculating mcg/min can be omitted.

EXAMPLE

Order: Infuse Heparin 10,000 U in 250 mL D5W at 0.4 U/kg/min

Weight: 59 kg

Drop Factor: 60 gtt/mL

1. How many U/min must be administered?

$$59 \text{ kg} \times \frac{0.4 \text{ U/min}}{1 \text{ kg}} = 23.6 \text{ U/min}$$

2. How many mL/hr will provide the required dose?

$$1 \text{ hr} \times \frac{60 \text{ min}}{1 \text{ hr}} \times \frac{23.6 \text{ U}}{1 \text{ min}} \times \frac{250 \text{ mL}}{10,000 \text{ U}} = 35 \text{ mL/hr}$$

3. How many gtt/min will provide the required dose?

$$1 \text{ min} \times \frac{23.6 \text{ U}}{1 \text{ min}} \times \frac{250 \text{ mL}}{10,000 \text{ U}} \times \frac{60 \text{ gtt}}{1 \text{ mL}} = 35 \text{ gtt/min}$$

OR

$$59 \text{ kg} \times \frac{0.4 \text{ U}}{1 \text{ kg}} \times \frac{250 \text{ mL}}{10,000 \text{ U}} \times \frac{60 \text{ gtt}}{1 \text{ mL}} = 35 \text{ gtt/min}$$

4. How many U/gtt will be administered?

$$1 \text{ gtt} \times \frac{1 \text{ min}}{35 \text{ gtt}} \times \frac{23.6 \text{ U}}{1 \text{ min}} = 0.7 \text{ U/gtt}$$

PRACTICE
IV Flow Rate and Dosages Based on Body Weight

1. **Order:** Infuse Amrinone 250 mg in 500 mL D5W at 5 mcg/kg/min
   Weight: 202 lb
   Drop Factor: 60 gtt/mL

   a. How many mcg/min must be administered?

   b. How many mL/hr will provide the required dose?

   c. How many gtt/min will provide the required dose?

   d. How many mcg/gtt will be administered?

2. **Order:** Infuse Dobutamine 250 mg in 250 mL D5W at 7 mcg/kg/min
   Weight: 73.6 kg
   Drop Factor: 60 gtt/mL

   a. How many mcg/min must be administered?

   b. How many mL/hr will provide the required dose?

   c. How many gtt/min will provide the required dose?

   d. How many mcg/gtt will be administered?

3. **Order:** Infuse Nitroprusside 50 mg in 250 mL D5W at 1.5 mcg/kg/min
   Weight: 198 lb
   Drop Factor: 60 gtt/mL

   a. How many mcg/min must be administered?

   b. How many mL/hr will provide the required dose?

   c. How many gtt/min will provide the required dose?

   d. How many mcg/gtt will be administered?

4. **Order:** Intropin (dopamine HCl) 800 mg in 250 mL D5W at 8 mcg/kg/min
   Weight: 72.8 kg
   Drop Factor: 60 gtt/mL

   a. How many mcg/min must be administered?

   b. How many mL/hr will provide the required dose?

   c. How many gtt/min will provide the require dose?

   d. How many mcg/gtt will be administered?

5. **Order:** Infuse Dobutamine 250 mg in 150 mL D5W at 5 mcg/kg/min
   Weight: 83.2 kg
   Drop Factor: 60 gtt/mL

   a. How many mcg/min must be administered?

   b. How many mL/hr will provide the required dose?

   c. How many gtt/min will provide the required dose?

   d. How many mcg/gtt will be administered?

(**Note:** See Appendix G for answer key.)

Titrated Infusions

Some very potent drugs are administered according to the patient's physiologic responses to the medication. That is, the dose is increased or decreased until the desired effect has been achieved. This effect may be: raising or lowering the blood pressure, controlling arrhythmias or seizures, relieving chest pain, or treating other often life-threatening situations.

The technique of adjusting dose/flow rate to obtain a precise desired effect is called *titration*. Examples of drugs administered by titration include: dopamine, nitroprusside, nitroglycerine, lidocaine, oxytocin, and magnesium sulfate.

Titrated drugs are given IV, either continuous or intermittent, depending on the volume and/or frequency of administration and equipment available. Small volume infusions may be administered via syringe or saline lock, and large volume infusions via an IV line, usually with a controlled volume set and always using an infusion pump.

Titration calculations are based on: solution concentration, infusion rate, and concentration of drug (i.e., mg/min, mcg/min, units/min, and mcg/kg/min). In addition, calculation of the *titration* (or *concentration*) *factor* (i.e., the concentration of drug per drop) (e.g., mg/gtt, μg/gtt, etc.) determines the exact amount of drug infusing any time a flow rate adjustment is made. The gtt/min may be increased or decreased depending on the patient's response to the current flow rate. The titration factor (drug/gtt) is used to determine the drug concentration (drug/min) provided by the adjusted flow rate.

Titrated drug orders may be written as a range of dosage between which the therapeutic dosage for an individual should fall (e.g., 5–10 mcg/kg/min). Therefore, the calculations involve determining the upper and lower therapeutic doses and titrating the dose within these limits. These calculations should be compared with the safe dose range recommended by the manufacturer.

Because titrated infusions require frequent dosage adjustments, it follows that the infusion pump settings must be readjusted simultaneously. Because of the minute changes in drug concentrations, it is essential that microdrip tubing be used. Therefore, the drop factor for calculating adjusted flow rates always will be 60 gtt/mL.

Several steps are necessary for calculating titrated infusions. Each step can be performed by using dimensional analysis, thus eliminating the need to memorize a confusing array of formulas. Each of the following steps has been presented in the preceding section; they are now arranged in the correct sequence for titration.

Steps in calculating titrated infusions:

1. Determine the concentration (drug/mL) of the solution to be administered.
2. Determine the amount of drug/min that will administer the ordered range of titration.
3. Determine how many mL/hr or gtt/min will administer the ordered range of titration.
4. Determine the titration (concentration) factor in drug/gtt.

5. If necessary, increase or decrease the gtt/min and determine the adjusted dosage (drug/min) the patient is receiving.

Continue titrating until the desired effect is achieved.

EXAMPLE

Order: Infuse Nipride (nitroprusside) 50 mg in 250 mL D5W. Titrate 3–6 mcg/kg/min to maintain the systolic blood pressure at 150 mm Hg

Weight: 135 lb

1. What is the concentration of the solution in mcg/mL?

Equivalents: 50 mg = 250 mL   1 mg = 1000 mcg

Conversion Equation:

$$1 \, \text{mL} \times \frac{50 \, \text{mg}}{250 \, \text{mL}} \times \frac{1000 \, \text{mcg}}{1 \, \text{mg}} = 200 \, \text{mcg/mL}$$

2. How many mcg/min will administer the ordered range of titration?

Lower (3 mcg/kg/min):

Equivalents: 1 kg = 2.2 lb   1 kg = 3 mcg/min

Conversion Equation:

$$135 \, \text{lb} \times \frac{1 \, \text{kg}}{2.2 \, \text{lb}} \times \frac{3 \, \text{mcg/min}}{1 \, \text{kg}} = 184 \, \text{mcg/min}$$

Upper (6 mcg/kg/min):

Equivalents: 1 kg = 2.2 lb   1 kg = 6 mcg/min

Conversion Equation:

$$135 \, \text{lb} \times \frac{1 \, \text{kg}}{2.2 \, \text{lb}} \times \frac{6 \, \text{mcg/min}}{1 \, \text{kg}} = 368 \, \text{mcg/min}$$

The range of dosage for this patient is 184–368 mcg/min.

3. How many mL/hr or gtt/min will administer the ordered range of titration?

Lower:

Equivalents: 1 hr = 60 min   1 min = 184 mcg
200 mcg = 1 mL

Conversion Equation:

$$1 \, \text{hr} \times \frac{60 \, \text{min}}{1 \, \text{hr}} \times \frac{184 \, \text{mcg}}{1 \, \text{min}} \times \frac{1 \, \text{mL}}{200 \, \text{mcg}} = 55 \, \text{mL/hr}$$

or 55 gtt/min

Upper:

Equivalents: 1 hr = 60 min 1 min = 368 mcg/min
200 mcg = 1 mL

Conversion Equation:

$$1\,hr \times \frac{60\,min}{1\,hr} \times \frac{368\,mcg}{1\,min} \times \frac{1\,mL}{200\,mcg}$$

$$= 110\ mL/hr\ or\ 110\ gtt/min$$

The range of mL/hr and gtt/min for this IV is 55–110 mL/hr or 55–110 gtt/min.

4. What is the titration (concentration) factor in mcg/gtt?

Equivalents: 55 gtt = 1 min 184 mcg = 1 min

Conversion Equation:

$$1\,gtt \times \frac{1\,min}{55\,gtt} \times \frac{184\,mcg}{1\,min} = 3.3\ mcg/gtt$$

5. The present systolic blood pressure reading is 170 mm Hg. Increase the gtt/min by 5 gtt. How many mcg/min will the patient now be receiving?

Equivalents: 1 min = 60 gtt 1 gtt = 3.3 mcg

Conversion Equation:

$$1\,min \times \frac{60\,gtt}{1\,min} \times \frac{3.3\,mcg}{1\,gtt} = 198\ mcg/min$$

6. After 1 hr, the systolic blood pressure reading is 120 mm Hg. Decrease the gtt/min by 6 gtt. How many mcg/min will the patient now be receiving?

Equivalents: 1 min = 54 gtt 1 gtt = 3.3 mcg

Conversion Equation:

$$1\,min \times \frac{54\,gtt}{1\,min} \times \frac{3.3\,mcg}{1\,gtt} = 178.2\ mcg/min$$

PRACTICE
Titration Infusions

1. **Order:** Infuse Esmolol HCl 5 g in 500 mL D5W. Titrate 50–100 mcg/kg/min to maintain the systolic blood pressure at 120 mm Hg. Weight: 140 lb

   a. What is the concentration of the solution in mcg/mL?

    b. How many mcg/min will administer the ordered range of titration?
Lower (50 mcg/kg/min):

    Upper (100 mcg/kg/min):

    c. How many mL/hr or gtt/min will administer the ordered range of titration?

    Lower:

    Upper:

    d. What is the titration (concentration) factor in mcg/gtt?

    e. The present systolic blood pressure reading is 160 mm Hg. Increase the gtt/min by 5 gtt. How many mcg/min will the patient now be receiving?

2. **Order:** Infuse Dopamine 400 mg in 500 mL D5W. Titrate 5–10 mcg/kg/min to maintain the systolic blood pressure greater than 100 mm Hg.
Weight: 175 lb

    a. What is the concentration of the solution in mcg/mL?

    b. How many mcg/min will administer the ordered range of titration?

Lower (5 mcg/kg/min):

Upper (10 mcg/kg/min):

c. How many mL/hr or gtt/min will administer the ordered range of titration?

Lower:

Upper:

d. What is the titration (concentration) factor in mcg/gtt?

e. The present systolic blood pressure reading is 68 mm Hg. Increase the gtt/min by 10 gtt. How many mcg/min will the patient now be receiving?

3. **Order:** Infuse Amrinone lactate 250 mg in 50 mL NS. Titrate 5–10 mcg/kg/min to maintain the diastolic blood pressure below 90 mm Hg.
   Weight: 70 kg

   a. What is the concentration of the solution in mcg/mL?

   b. How many mcg/min will administer the ordered range of titration?

Lower (5 mcg/kg/min):

Upper (10 mcg/kg/min):

c. How many mL/hr or gtt/min will administer the ordered range of titration?

Lower:

Upper:

d. What is the titration (concentration) factor in mcg/gtt?

e. The present diastolic blood pressure reading is 100 mm Hg. Increase the gtt/min by 5 gtt. How many mcg/min will the patient now be receiving?

4. **Order:** Infuse Nitropress (nitroprusside sodium) 50 mg in 500 mL D5W. Titrate 1.5–3 mcg/kg/min to maintain the systolic blood pressure at 100 mm Hg.
Weight: 200 lb

a. What is the concentration of the solution in mcg/mL?

    b. How many mcg/min will administer the ordered range of titration?

        Lower (1.5 mcg/kg/min):

        Upper (3 mcg/kg/min):

    c. How many mL/hr or gtt/min will administer the ordered range of titration?

        Lower:

        Upper:

    d. What is the titration (concentration) factor in mcg/gtt?

    e. The present systolic blood pressure reading is 90 mm Hg. Decrease the gtt/min by 5 gtt. How many mcg/min will the patient now be receiving?

5. **Order:** Infuse Dopamine Hydrochloride 200 mg in 500 mL D5W. Titrate 2–5 mcg/kg/min to maintain the systolic blood pressure at a minimum of 100 mm Hg.
   Weight: 165 lb

    a. What is the concentration of the solution in mcg/mL?

    b. How many mcg/min will administer the ordered range of titration?

Lower (2 mcg/kg/min):

Upper (5 mcg/kg/min):

c. How many mL/hr or gtt/min will administer the ordered range of titration?

Lower:

Upper:

d. What is the titration (concentration) factor in mcg/gtt?

e. The present systolic blood pressure reading is 80 mm Hg. Increase the gtt/min by 5 gtt. How many mcg/min will the patient now be receiving?

(**Note:** See Appendix G for answer key.)

Drugs Administered by IV Bolus

When a small amount of medication is injected directly into a vein, it is called an IV bolus or IV push. A venipuncture can be performed in any accessible vein and the medication injected by means of a syringe. If an IV is already in place, the medication can be injected through a Y-port or the flashball at the end of the infusion tubing. An IV bolus also can be given through the saline lock. Some infusion pumps are designed to deliver an IV bolus at a controlled rate.

Because drugs given by IV bolus will have an immediate effect, the rate of injection becomes extremely important. Administering IV injections too quickly can result in adverse side effects and/or speed shock. Many drugs are ordered to be injected over a period of 1–30 minutes. On the other hand, some drugs must be given rapidly, even within a period of seconds, because an immediate effect is desired or necessary. It is, therefore, essential to determine the correct IV injection rate and to time this accurately using a clock or wristwatch with a second hand. The need for precision in this regard cannot be overemphasized.

EXAMPLE   **Order:** Chloromycetin 300 mg IV bolus via saline lock

Label: Chloromycetin (chloramphenicol) 1 g

Directions: Reconstitute with 10 mL sterile water for injection to yield 100 mg/mL. Safe injection rate is 1 g/min.

a. How many mL of Chloromycetin should be administered?

Equivalents: 1 g = 10 mL   1000 mg = 1 g

Conversion Equation:

$$300 \text{ mg} \times \frac{1 \text{ g}}{1000 \text{ mg}} \times \frac{10 \text{ mL}}{1 \text{ g}} = 3 \text{ mL}$$

b. How long should it take to administer this IV bolus?

Equivalents: 1 g = 10 mL   1000 mg = 1 g

Conversion Equation:

$$3 \text{ mL} \times \frac{1 \text{ g}}{10 \text{ mL}} \times \frac{1 \text{ min}}{1 \text{ g}} = 0.3 \text{ min} = 18 \text{ seconds}$$

OR

$$300 \text{ mg} \times \frac{1 \text{ g}}{1000 \text{ mg}} \times \frac{1 \text{ min}}{1 \text{ g}} = 0.3 \text{ min} = 18 \text{ seconds}$$

PRACTICE
IV Bolus

1. **Order:** Emete-Con 20 mg IV bolus via 3-way stopcock of infusion tubing
   Label: Emete-Con 50 mg
   Directions: Reconstitute with 2.2 mL of sterile water for injection to yield a concentration of 25 mg/mL. Safe injection rate is 25 mg/30 sec. (The apparent discrepancy here between amount of added diluent

and amount of resulting solution is explained by the *hydrophilic* property of Emete-Con, i.e., possessing the ability to absorb moisture.)

   a. How many mL should be injected?

   b. How long should it take to administer this IV bolus?

FIGURE 10-21

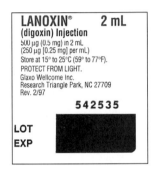

LANOXIN®   **2 mL**
(digoxin) Injection
500 µg (0.5 mg) in 2 mL
(250 µg [0.25 mg] per mL)
Store at 15° to 25°C (59° to 77°F).
PROTECT FROM LIGHT.
Glaxo Wellcome Inc.
Research Triangle Park, NC 27709
Rev. 2/97

542535

LOT
EXP

2. Order: Digoxin 0.5 mg IV bolus via primary infusion line
   Label: Figure 10-21
   Directions: Do not exceed rate of 0.25 mg/min for IV bolus.

   a. How many mL of Digoxin should be administered?

   b. What is the least number of minutes it should take to administer this IV bolus of Digoxin?

FIGURE 10-22

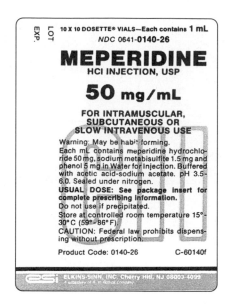

3. **Order:** Demerol 30 mg IV bolus via Y-tube/primary line
   Label: Figure 10-22
   Directions: Do not exceed rate of 25 mg/min for IV bolus.

   a. What is the total amount of solution to be injected?

   b. How long should it take to administer this IV bolus?

FIGURE 10-23

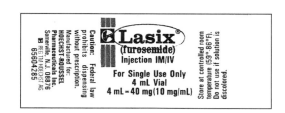

4. **Order:** Lasix 35 mg IV bolus via saline lock
   Label: Figure 10-23
   Directions: Administer undiluted. Maximum injection rate = 20 mg/min.

   a. What is the total amount of solution to be injected?

   b. How long should it take to administer this IV bolus?

5. **Order:** Aminophylline 240 mg IV bolus via saline lock
   Label: Aminophylline 25 mg/mL
   Directions: Do not exceed rate of 25 mg/min for IV bolus.

      a. How many mL of Aminophylline should be administered?

      b. What is the least number of minutes required to administer this IV bolus of Aminophylline into the saline lock?

6. **Order:** Bretylium 5 mg/kg IV bolus
   Label: Bretylium 500 mg/mL
   Directions: Do not exceed injection rate of 25 mg/min.

      a. How many mg should be administered via bolus (patient weighs 135 lb)?

      b. How many mL would the bolus contain?

      c. How long should it take to administer this bolus?

7. **Order:** Lidocaine 1 mg/kg IV bolus. Follow by Lidocaine drip 1000 mg/250 mL of D5W and run at 2 mg/min.
   Label: Bolus-Lidocaine (1%) 10 mg/mL
   Label: IV-Lidocaine (20%) 200 mg/mL
   Directions: Do not exceed injection rate of 35 mg/min.

      a. How many mg of Lidocaine (1%) would be administered via bolus (patient weighs 170 lb)?

b. How many mL would the bolus contain?

c. How long should it take to administer this bolus?

d. How many mL of Lidocaine (20%) should be added to the IV?

e. How many mL/hr should be administered IV?

(**Note:** See Appendix G for answer key.)

Parenteral Nutrition   When nutritional needs cannot be met by enteral intake, supplementary or total nutrition can be provided via parenteral routes. Basic nutrients, electrolytes, and vitamins, as well as fluid requirements, can be administered intravenously through a peripheral or central vein. Choice of route depends on tonicity and/or concentration of the solution, as well as anticipated duration of parenteral nutrition administration.

Terms associated with parenteral nutrition include:

TPN: total parenteral nutrition—all nutrients essential for tissue maintenance are provided intravenously.

CPN: refers to IV nutrition via a central vein, usually the superior vena cava. The terms TPN and CPN often are used interchangeably.

PTPN: peripheral total parenteral nutrition (or PPN—peripheral parenteral nutrition) refers to IV nutrition via a peripheral vein, usually the radial, basilic, or cephalic vein of the arm.

Hyperalimentation: refers to the provision of nutrients in excess of maintenance needs.

Regardless of the route used for administration, it is important to remember that parenteral nutrition solutions are natural culture mediums for bacterial growth and should not hang in excess of 12 hr.

Nutrition calculations can be used to determine the amounts of nutrients and energy contained in a parenteral nutrition formula (IV solution).

Generally, they are concerned with the caloric value, expressed as kilocalories (kcal) of the glucose, amino acid, and/or fat emulsion content of the IV solution.

Equivalents necessary for setting up the conversion equations include:

*1 g glucose = 3.4 kcal

1 g amino acid (protein) = 4 kcal

1 g of 10% fat emulsion = 1.1 kcal

1 g of 20% fat emulsion = 2 kcal

In a percentage solution, the symbol % refers to *parts of substance (solid) per 100 parts of solution* (liquid) (i.e., 1 g of solid is equivalent to 1 mL of liquid). See Appendix F, Percentage Solutions: Equivalent Units for Solids and Liquids.

Thus: a 5% solution indicates 5 g/100 mL

a 2.5% solution indicates 2.5 g/100 mL

*Note: kcal values for intravenous CHO and fat are different from the kcal values for the same orally ingested nutrients. Protein values are unchanged.

4 kcal/g of CHO

4 kcal/g of protein

9 kcal/g of fat

EXAMPLE   **Order:** TPN 1000 mL D5W (carbohydrate), 500 mL Liposyn II 10% (fat), 500 mL Aminosyn 3.5% (protein) IV

How many kcal of carbohydrates, fats, and proteins are provided by this IV?

Carbohydrates:

Equivalents: 5 g = 100 mL   1 g = 3.4 kcal

Conversion Equation:

$$1000 \; mL \times \frac{5 \; g}{100 \; mL} \times \frac{3.4 \; kcal}{1 \; g} = 170 \; kcal$$

Fats:

Equivalents: 10 g = 100 mL   1 g = 1.1 kcal

Conversion Equation:

$$500 \; mL \times \frac{10 \; g}{100 \; mL} \times \frac{1.1 \; kcal}{1 \; g} = 55 \; kcal$$

Protein:

Equivalents: 3.5 g = 100 mL   1 g = 4 kcal

Conversion Equation:

$$500 \; mL \times \frac{3.5 \; g}{100 \; mL} \times \frac{4 \; kcal}{1 \; g} = 70 \; kcal$$

PRACTICE
Nutrition Calculations

1. **Order:** TPN 1500 mL D5W IV
   How many kcal of carbohydrate are provided?

2. **Order:** TPN 1000 mL Aminosyn 3.5% IV
   How many kcal of protein are provided?

3. **Order:** CPN 1000 mL Liposyn II 10% IV
   How many kcal of fat are provided?

4. **Order:** TPN 500 mL 2.5% Dextrose in Water IV
   How many kcal of carbohydrate are provided?

5. **Order:** PTPN 1500 mL Aminosyn PF 7% IV
   How many kcal of protein are provided?

6. **Order:** TPN 2500 mL D10W IV
   How many kcal of carbohydrate are provided?

7. **Order:** CPN 1500 mL Intralipid 20% IV
   How many kcal of fat are provided?

8. **Order:** TPN 3000 mL 20% Dextrose in Water IV
   How many kcal of carbohydrate are provided?

9. **Order:** TPN 1000 mL Aminosyn II 5% and 500 mL 25% Dextrose in Water IV

   a. How many kcal of protein are provided?

   b. How many kcal of carbohydrates are provided?

10. **Order:** TPN 1000 mL Aminosyn II 4.25% and 1000 mL D10W IV

    a. How many kcal of protein are provided?

    b. How many kcal of carbohydrate are provided?

(**Note:** See Appendix G for answer key.)

Assessment and Adjustment

One of the major responsibilities of the nurse who is caring for patients with intravenous infusions is observation and assessment. The flow rate is assessed by counting the drops per minute (gtt/min) and determining what adjustments need to be made in the event the rate has changed. A checklist, such as the example in Figure 10-24, may be useful in performing the IV assessment.

A variety of factors can affect the flow rate including positional changes that may alter the angle of the needle or catheter, a clot that partially obstructs the infusion flow, improper height of the container, tubing dangling below insertion site, dislodgement of needle or clamp, and infiltration or irritation at the insertion site.

Regardless of the infusion system used (e.g., gravity [infusion], controller, or pump), nursing assessment is of prime importance, because early observation and correction of undesirable factors are essential to maintain the infusion at the designated rate and to prevent adverse occurrences. Even if the IV is attached to an automatic infusion pump or controller, frequent observation is necessary to be sure the system is working properly and the desired flow rate is being maintained.

Although the previous section dealt with the use of dimensional analysis to calculate the initial flow rate, most nurses will be much more frequently involved with maintaining IV infusions than starting them. This involves periodic observation of the amount of fluid remaining to be infused and recalculation of the flow rate to determine if adjustments need to be made to complete the IV within the ordered time period. Dimensional analysis lends itself equally well to determining the need for adjustment of the flow rate when any of the previously mentioned factors have caused it to speed up or slow down.

FIGURE 10-24
IV assessment

IV ASSESSMENT

Pt. Initials _____ Room # _____

Name of IV fluid being infused _____

_____

#mL left in bag/bottle _____

Flow rate: _____ cc/hr or _____ gtt/min

Without disturbing dressing, what is condition of IV site? _____

_____

What time do you anticipate IV bag/bottle will need to be changed? _____

What IV solution will be hung next? _____

EXAMPLE ■ **Starting IV**

Order: 1000 mL of Sodium Chloride 0.9% to infuse over a period of 8 hr.

Drop Factor: 15 gtt/mL

Question: What should the flow rate be when the IV is started?

Answer:

$$1 \text{ min} \times \frac{1 \text{ hr}}{60 \text{ min}} \times \frac{1000 \text{ mL}}{8 \text{ hr}} \times \frac{15 \text{ gtt}}{1 \text{ mL}} = 31 \text{ gtt}$$

■ **Assessing the IV**

After the IV has been running 5 hr, there are still 450 mL left to infuse. Does the IV flow rate need to be adjusted to complete the infusion in the ordered time period?

Two factors must be noted in this problem. First, the total amount of solution is now 450 mL; second, the total number of hours remaining is 3.

The conversion equation is written exactly as before, substituting the new values in the conversion factor mL/hr.

$$1 \text{ min} \times \frac{1 \text{ hr}}{60 \text{ min}} \times \frac{450 \text{ mL}}{3 \text{ hr}} \times \frac{15 \text{ gtt}}{1 \text{ mL}} = 37.5 = 38 \text{ gtt}$$

■ **Adjusting the IV**

The IV flow rate must be adjusted to 38 gtt/min.

REMEMBER

Although minor adjustments in flow rate are permissible (usually less than 25% increase over the initial flow rate), larger increases require a physician's order. One exception is in the administration of parenteral nutrition when any flow rate increase could be hazardous. Whenever there is a question, consult the physician.

PRACTICE
Adjusting IVs (Calculate in gtt/min)

1. **Order:** 2500 mL of D5W IV to infuse over a period of 12 hr
   Drop Factor: 10 gtt/mL

   a. What should the flow rate be when the IV is started?

b. After the IV has been running 8 hours, there are still 800 mL left to infuse. To what should the flow rate be adjusted to have the IV completed on schedule?

2. **Order:** 1000 mL Lactated Ringers IV in 6 hr
   Drop Factor: 15 gtt/mL

   a. What should the initial flow rate be?

   b. After 4 hr, 350 mL remain. To what should the flow rate be adjusted to have the IV completed on schedule?

3. **Order:** 3000 mL D5W IV in 24 hr
   Drop Factor: 20 gtt/mL

   a. What should the initial flow rate be?

   b. After 18 hr, 600 mL remain. What should the adjusted flow rate be?

4. **Order:** 1500 mL D2.5W IV in 12 hr
   Drop Factor: 10 gtt/mL

   a. What should the initial flow rate be?

   b. After 7 hr, 800 mL remain. What should the adjusted flow rate be?

5. **Order:** 500 mL Sodium Chloride 0.9% IV in 8 hr
   Drop Factor: 60 gtt/mL

   a. What should the initial flow rate be?

    b. After 5 hr, 150 mL remain. What should the adjusted flow rate be?

6. **Order:** 750 mL Ringers IV in 4 hr
   Drop Factor: 10 gtt/mL

    a. What should the initial flow rate be?

    b. After 2½ hr, 300 mL remain. What should the adjusted flow rate be?

7. **Order:** 2000 mL D5W IV in 18 hr
   Drop Factor: 15 gtt/mL

    a. What should the initial flow rate be?

    b. After 11 hr, 900 mL remain. What should the adjusted flow rate be?

8. **Order:** 250 mL Isolyte M IV in 5 hr
   Drop Factor: 60 gtt/mL

    a. What should the initial flow rate be?

    b. After 2 hr, 120 mL remain. What should the adjusted flow rate be?

9. **Order:** 1250 mL D2.5NS IV in 9 hr
   Drop Factor: 15 gtt/mL

    a. What should the initial flow rate be?

b. After 3 hr, 750 mL remain. What should the adjusted flow rate be?

10. **Order:** 125 mL Sodium Chloride 0.9% in 2 hr IV
   Drop Factor: 60 gtt/mL

   a. What should the initial flow rate be?

   b. After 1½ hr, 30 mL remain. What should the adjusted flow rate be?

(**Note:** See Appendix G for answer key.)

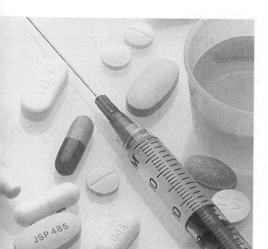

CHAPTER 11

Administration of Intravenous Medications and Solutions

OBJECTIVES

Upon completion of this chapter you should be able to:

- Identify safe and suitable sites for intravenous injections and infusions.
- Identify nursing responsibilities in relation to administering, assessing, and monitoring intravenous injections and infusions.
- Follow infection-control guidelines with respect to safe handling or manipulation of IV equipment.
- Identify performance criteria related to IV medications and solutions.

Intravenous Administration

A variety of methods can be used when medications or fluids are given intravenously. The traditional method has been the gravity infusion system. This method, commonly referred to as "an IV," is called a continuous infusion and is employed for the purpose of providing or replacing fluids directly into the blood, rather than via the gastrointestinal route. Medications can be added to this continuous IV for slow administration or can be infused directly into the intravenous line for more rapid administration. The latter is called intermittent infusion and may be administered via IV piggy back, a volume control set, a saline lock, or a central venous catheter; medications also can be injected directly into a vein by means of an IV bolus (push).

Although nurses increasingly are assuming responsibility for starting IVs and administering IV medications, these activities require specialized knowledge and are regulated by nurse practice acts and agency policy. Nurses should be aware of their professional and legal responsibilities with respect to intravenous administration.

Infusion Sites

Any easily accessible vein may be chosen for venipuncture. Most commonly used are the hand and lower arm, the antecubital fossa, and the upper arm, Figure 11-1. Less desirable are veins in the legs and feet, because of the greater risk of thrombophlebitis and embolism. A central venous line may be used for infusion directly through a major vein such as the subclavian. In infants, a scalp vein often is used.

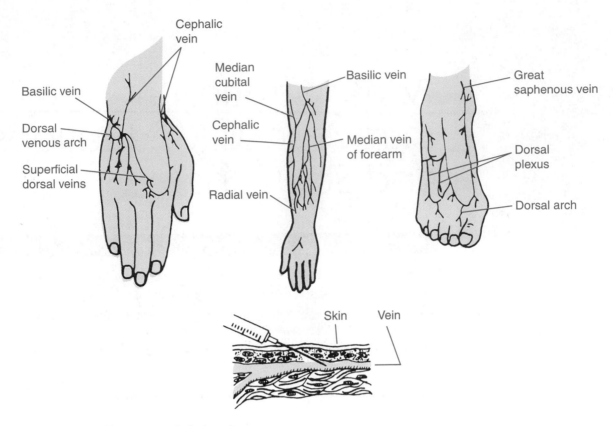

FIGURE 11-1   Intravenous infusion sites

When veins are inaccessible or very difficult to reach, a venisection may be required. In this procedure, called a cut-down, the skin is incised to expose a vein for insertion of the IV needle.

Nursing Responsibilities Relative to Intravenous Administration

In addition to the principles for administration of medications listed in Chapters 7 and 9, specific nursing responsibilities in relation to intravenous injections and infusions include the following:

- Setting up for an intravenous infusion: obtaining correct solution, infusion set, and needle; attaching and priming tubing; adding medication if ordered; and labeling container appropriately (e.g., patient's name, solution, rate, date, and time). Felt tip pens should never be used to label IV bags as the ink can leak through the plastic and contaminate the solution.

- Positioning patient comfortably, explaining procedure, preparing venipuncture site: shaving, immobilizing, etc.

- Performing venipuncture, initiating intravenous infusion, adjusting flow rate, and terminating infusion upon completion.

- Monitoring the intravenous infusion by maintaining flow rate as ordered. The rate of flow should be checked by counting the number of drops per minute at least every 30 min or more often if necessary, even if an IV pump or controller is in use. If this is done, the ordered flow rate can be maintained with very minor adjustments being required. It is important to keep in mind the risks associated with too slow or too rapid administration of intravenous solutions. (**Note:** The flow rate may be checked by counting the drop rate for 15 sec and multiplying by 4.)

■ Checking patency of the system, placement of needle or intracatheter and condition of site; attaching additional containers of fluid as ordered; noting and recording amount of fluid administered.

■ Administering medication through the IV.

■ Changing IV dressing and/or IV tubing as necessary or according to hospital policy.

■ Providing physical care for the patient including assistance with meals, ambulation, comfort, and hygiene.

■ Observing for complications associated with intravenous administration:

1. Fluid overload resulting from too rapid administration of intravenous solutions.

   Signs: rapid breathing

   shortness of breath

   dilation of neck veins

   increase in blood pressure

   decreased fluid output in relation to fluid intake

2. Speed shock resulting from too rapid administration of intravenous medication, especially bolus injection.

   Signs: headache

   flushed face

   irregular pulse

   decrease in blood pressure (shock)

(**Note:** The nurse should use caution in increasing the IV flow rate even if it is running behind schedule. Speeding up the IV in an attempt to catch up and complete in the specified time could cause fluid overload or speed shock. If major adjustments in flow rate are deemed necessary, a physician's order should be obtained.)

3. Infiltration (leakage) of IV solution into subcutaneous tissue surrounding venipuncture site due to displacement of needle or intracatheter.

   Signs: sluggish flow rate

   absence of blood backflow

   localized swelling, pallor, pain

   area cool to touch

4. Thrombophlebitis (injury or irritation to a vein) resulting in clot formation at end of needle or intracatheter.

   Signs: sluggish flow rate

   pain or tenderness, redness, heat at IV site and/or along affected vein

5. Allergic reaction to IV fluid or additive.

>   Signs: rash
>
>   itching
>
>   shortness of breath

6. Infection at venipuncture site related to improper care of IV site (i.e., dressing changes, etc.).

>   Signs: discharge
>
>   inflammation

7. Systemic infection related to contamination of equipment or solutions.

>   Signs: elevated TPR
>
>   chills, malaise

8. Air embolism resulting from air in tubing due to loose connections or containers running dry. (**Note:** More common when an infusion pump is being used.)

>   Signs: cyanosis
>
>   hypotension
>
>   weak, rapid pulse
>
>   loss of consciousness

9. Catheter embolism resulting from improper insertion, accidental breakage, or dislodgement.

>   Signs: same as air embolism, plus discomfort in involved vein

Precautions in Handling IV Equipment

Because the administration of IV fluids and medications involves the risk of coming into contact with blood and/or body fluids, it is essential that:

- sterile technique be maintained in performing venipuncture, changing site dressings, and manipulating any equipment that subjects the patient to the risk of infection.

- personnel observe blood and body fluid precautions as recommended by the Centers for Disease Control. This includes wearing gloves when flushing lumens, starting and terminating IVs, or performing any procedure that subjects personnel to a risk of infection through contact with blood or body fluids.

- all needles used in administration of intravenous therapy be discarded into puncture-resistant containers.

Recording

Intravenous medications and solutions are recorded in a variety of locations depending on policies of the agency. These may include the MAR, a special intravenous form, nurses notes, and/or the intake/output record. The initial notation should include information relative to time, type, site, and flow rate. Subsequent notations document ongoing assessment, observations, flow rate, additives, patient's response, adverse effects, and time of termination.

**Performance Criteria:
Setting Up an IV**

The learner is referred to a nursing text or skills manual for detailed instruction on performance of venipuncture and administration of continuous intravenous infusion. The following checklists may be helpful as a guide for intravenous administration.

	S	U	Comments
1. Washes hands			
2. Gathers equipment **a)** Bottle or bag of prescribed IV solution			
b) Proper tubing (vented or nonvented)			
c) IV pole			
3. Examines the container **a)** Correct solution			
b) Correct amount			
c) Expiration date			
d) Glass bottle, intact			
e) Plastic bag (absence of dimples or puncture marks)			
f) Solution, clear			
4. Examines the tubing **a)** Spike cover, intact and secure			
5. Slides flow clamp along tubing until it is directly under drip chamber and closes the clamp			
6. Spikes the container **a)** Bottle with rubber stopper (uses vented tubing). Removes metal cap, swabs stopper with alcohol; places bottle on stable surface, steadies by holding stopper between finger and thumb; removes plastic cover from spike and pushes spike firmly into rubber stopper, avoiding contamination; hangs on IV pole			

Continues

	S	U	Comments
b) Bottle with indwelling vent and a latex diaphragm (uses nonvented tubing). Removes protective metal cap and diaphragm; notes release of vacuum; inserts spike in proper opening; hangs on IV pole			
c) Plastic bag (uses nonvented tubing). Hangs on IV pole before spiking; steadies port with one hand and removes protective cap by pulling smoothly to the right; inserts spike into port with one quick motion			
7. Gently squeezes drip chamber until half full (or full, depending on equipment instructions)			
8. Primes the tubing **a)** Holds end over sink, wastebasket, etc.			
b) Removes protective cap, without contaminating inside (does not discard cap)			
c) Unclamps tubing and lets fluid run through until it fills the tubing and all air bubbles have been expelled. Maintains sterility of end of tubing			
d) If small bubbles appear at top of tubing or in drip chamber, lightly taps area until bubbles rise into chamber			
e) Clamps off tubing and replaces protective cap			
9. Loops tubing over IV pole until ready to perform venipuncture			
10. Labels container and tubing with date, time of insertion and any medication added			

S—Satisfactory   U—Unsatisfactory   Evaluator _____

**Performance Criteria:
Starting IV (with an
Over-the-Needle Type
Catheter)**

	S	U	Comments
1. Washes hands			
2. Obtains equipment and sets up IV			
3. Prepares patient for procedure			
4. Selects vein; shaves site if necessary			
5. Applies tourniquet			
6. Puts on gloves			
7. Preps insertion site with antiseptic			
8. Removes protective shield from catheter set			
9. Grasps patient's arm so that the thumb below the insertion site increases skin tension and stabilizes the vein			
10. Places needle at 30° angle with bevel up, about 1 cm distal to venipuncture site			
11. Punctures the skin so that the needle approaches the vein from the side			
12. Advances the needle into the vein at a slight angle to the vein, with slow, steady pressure			
13. Aligns the needle with the vein and follows the vein until about an eighth of an inch of the plastic catheter is within the lumen			
14. After blood flows into the body of the catheter releases thumb pressure on patient's arm, holds the metal needle firmly in place with one hand and advances the plastic catheter smoothly into the vein			
15. Continues to advance the catheter until the catheter hub is approximately one-fourth inch from the puncture site			

Continues

	S	U	Comments
16. Loosens the tourniquet, holds the catheter steady, withdraws and discards metal needle into puncture-resistant container as soon as possible			
17. Removes cap from the IV tubing and joins the catheter and tubing adapters firmly together			
18. Opens the clamp on the IV tubing to a fast rate to check for free-flow, then partially closes clamp			
19. Tapes the catheter hub to the patient's arm			
20. Applies dressing in such a manner that dressing can be changed without disturbing the catheter			
21. Forms a loose loop in the tubing and tapes to patient's arm			
22. Adjusts the IV flow to the prescribed rate			
23. Indicates the size of the needle and date on the tape			
24. Secures an armboard in such a manner that circulation and comfort are not impaired			

S—Satisfactory   U—Unsatisfactory   Evaluator _____

Performance Criteria: Assessment, Adjustment, and Termination of IV

	S	U	Comments
1. Assesses by observing			
a) patency of tubing			
b) rate of flow			
c) amount remaining			
d) injection site			
e) patient's reaction			
2. Adjusts flow rate to correct number of drops/minute			

	S	U	Comments
3. Terminates when indicated, applying principles of asepsis, safety, and comfort **a)** puts on gloves			
b) clamps off			
c) loosens tape			
d) places sterile gauze pad over site			
e) withdraws needle, immediately applies pressure and elevates limb			
f) discards needle into puncture-resistant container			
g) maintains pressure as necessary			
h) applies Band-Aid securely			

S—Satisfactory   U—Unsatisfactory   Evaluator _____

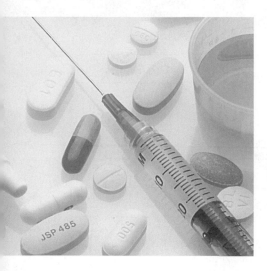

CHAPTER 12

Pediatric Dosage

OBJECTIVES

Upon completion of this chapter you should be able to:

- Identify special considerations related to safety and comfort when administering medications to infants and children.
- Identify adaptations and special considerations related to administration of oral and parenteral medications to infants and children when giving intramuscular injections and intravenous infusions.
- Apply dimensional analysis to clinical calculations of pediatric dosage based on body weight and body surface area.

There are several methods for calculating pediatric medication dosage based on various combinations of age, height, weight, body surface area, and adult dose. Because children of the same age can vary widely in size and weight, many of the usual methods are not applicable in all cases. Furthermore, rules or formulas do not take into consideration the physical condition of the child and the variety of responses and/or susceptibilities to the effects of drugs possible in individual children. Because of the serious consequences that may result from overdosage or underdosage, accuracy of calculating and precision of administering medications to infants and children is of prime importance.

General Considerations in Administering Oral and Parenteral Medications to Children

- Be sure positive identification has been made by comparison of name tag with medication administration guide or other means. Do not rely on child's response to spoken name.
- Corroborate calculated dosages by double-checking with another nurse and/or referring to a drug information source. This is particularly important when administering insulin, heparin, or digoxin.
- Exercise particular caution in maintaining security of drugs, medication cart, needles, syringes, etc., making sure they are not accessible to children.
- Be sure child is awake and alert before administering oral medications. Never administer oral medications to a crying or resisting child or an injection to a sleeping child.
- Make explanations according to child's developmental level of understanding regarding reasons for medication, route of administration, expected sensations, taste, etc. Allow child to express feelings; be accepting of negative reactions.
- Maintain a firm, but friendly manner. Give praise and comfort following administration.

- Restrain child gently, but firmly. Obtain assistance as necessary, particularly for injections.

- Children up to 3 years of age are unable to swallow pills, and even older children may have much difficulty. Crush and dissolve pills and tablets (exclusive of enteric coated) as necessary. Administer liquids via cup, spoon, dropper, or syringe. For infants, medications can be placed in an empty nipple, from which the infant can suck.

Administration of Parenteral Medications to Infants and Children

Intramuscular Injections

The site of choice for intramuscular injections in infants and children under the age of 3 is the lateral aspect of the thigh, the vastus lateralis muscle. The reason for this is that in children under the age of 3 years, the gluteal muscle is very small and poorly developed, and injection in this area is dangerously close to the sciatic nerve. The vastus lateralis site is located by measuring two to three finger breadths above the knee and below the trochanter depending on the size of the child.

The ventrogluteal site is acceptable in children over 3 years who have been walking for 1 year or more, and is a good site because it is free of major nerves and blood vessels. Figure 12-1 illustrates the method for locating this site. The thumb is placed on the anterior superior iliac spine and the index finger is abducted posteriorly. The injection site is located between the thumb and index finger. The dorsogluteal site should be avoided until the child is over age 4.

In older children, over age 5, the deltoid muscle is an acceptable site as long as the number and volume of injections is limited.

For any of the IM sites, volume of injections should be limited to a maximum of:

1 mL—birth to 5 years

2 mL—6 to 12 years

FIGURE 12-1
Ventrogluteal site in child

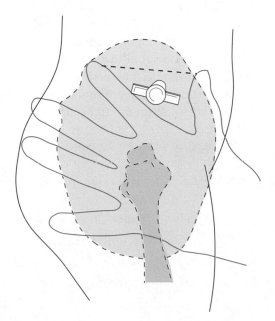

Special consideration must be given to safety aspects of administering injections. Needles with a smaller diameter and shorter length should be used. For most infants and small children, a 25 gauge, 1″ needle is preferable unless solution is too viscous. Children must be restrained to avoid injury. A mummy restraint is suitable for infants; older children can be gently, but firmly restrained by the person giving the injection or by another individual, if necessary. Make explanations brief, give injections quickly but safely, and allow the child to cry or express feelings. It is especially important for the nurse or parent to pick up, soothe, and comfort infants and young children following an injection.

Intravenous Infusions

Because infants have such small arm and hand veins, scalp veins (temporal area) or the superior longitudinal sinus often are chosen as intravenous sites. In young children, the external jugular vein is an acceptable alternative site. When a scalp vein is used, the area must be shaved. It is important to avoid cuts during shaving, because of the danger of infection. A scalp vein needle is securely taped in place and covered with a gauze dressing. Additional protection such as a small plastic or paper cup is necessary to prevent dislodgement.

In young children, acceptable intravenous sites are the veins on the dorsal surface of the hand or flexor surface of the wrist; also the leg and foot veins. The antecubital site is used least often, because of the difficulty of preventing dislodgement.

Infants and young children must be restrained adequately during insertion of the needle and the duration of the infusion. Mummy and/or elbow restraints and sandbags are effective methods. Armboards or other immobilizing devices may be used for older children.

Intravenous infusions must be checked as often as every 15–30 minutes. Because of the greater risk of fluid overload, an automatic rate-flow infusion pump always should be used to regulate and maintain the rate of flow. A pediatric infusion set featuring volume control is an additional safety measure to prevent IV fluid overload by allowing only 50–100 mL of solution into the fluid chamber at one time. The minidrip feature of the volume control infusion set allows for easier regulation of the flow rate and more precise intravenous administration. A syringe-pump (mini-infuser) is useful in administering small amounts of intravenous fluids at a controlled rate. It is essential to maintain an accurate record of fluid intake and output on children receiving IV infusions. The 5% rule should be observed in pediatric as well as adult IV Therapy.

Pediatric Dosage Based on Body Weight—Oral Medications

EXAMPLE

Order: Digoxin Elixir Pediatric 15 mcg/kg of body weight/dose po

Label: Digoxin 0.05 mg/mL

Weight: 60 lb

How many mL should the child receive per dose?

Starting Factor	Answer Unit
60 lb	mL

Equivalents: 1 kg = 2.2 lb   15 mcg = 1 kg
1000 mcg (μg) = 1 mg 0.05 mg = 1 mL

Conversion Equation:

$$60\,\text{lb} \times \frac{1\,\text{kg}}{2.2\,\text{lb}} \times \frac{15\,\text{mcg}}{1\,\text{kg}} \times \frac{1\,\text{mg}}{1000\,\text{mcg}} \times \frac{1\,\text{mL}}{0.05\,\text{mg}} = 8.2\,\text{mL}$$

EXAMPLE

Order: Coly-Mycin S 5 mg/kg of body weight/day po to be given in 3 divided doses

Label: Coly-Mycin S (Colestimethate sodium) 25 mg/5 mL

Weight: 4.5 kg

How many drops should be administered per dose?

Equivalents: 25 mg = 5 mL, 5 mg = 1 kg, 15 gtt = 1 mL, 3 doses - 4.5 kg

Conversion Equation:

$$4.5\,\text{kg} \times \frac{5\,\text{mg}}{1\,\text{kg}} \times \frac{5\,\text{mL}}{25\,\text{mg}} \times \frac{15\,\text{gtt}}{1\,\text{mL}} = \frac{67.5\,\text{gtt}}{3\,\text{doses}} = 22.5 = 23\,\text{gtt}$$

Because it is important to administer the exact amount ordered, the computation should be carried out to two decimal places and rounded to the nearest tenth. To obtain a more precise measurement than is possible with a medicine cup, the medication should be measured using a syringe. It then may be administered directly from the syringe.

PRACTICE
Calculating Pediatric Dosage Based on Body Weight—Oral Medications

1. **Order:** Lanoxin Elixir 30 μg/kg/dose po
   Label: Figure 12-2. What is the generic name? _____
   Weight: 28 lb
   How many mL should the child receive?

FIGURE 12-2

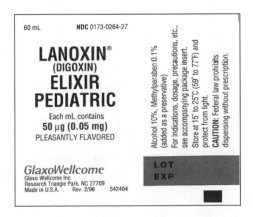

2. **Order:** Amoxicillin Suspension 20 mg/kg in three divided doses/day po
   Label: Figure 12-3
   Weight: 44 lb
   How many mL should be administered per dose?

FIGURE 12-3

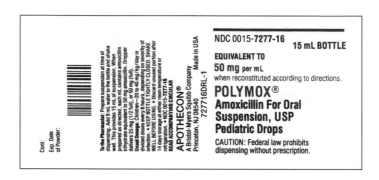

3. **Order:** Cefaclor Oral Suspension 40 mg/kg/day in 3 divided doses po
   Label: Figure 12-4
   Weight: 40 lb
   How many mL should be administered per dose?

FIGURE 12-4

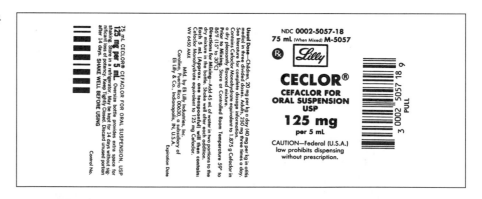

4. **Order:** Gantrisin Pediatric Suspension 150 mg/kg po in four divided doses/day
   Label: Gantrisin Pediatric Suspension (sulfasoxizole) 0.5 g/tsp
   Weight: 40 lb
   How many mL should be administered per dose?

5. **Order:** Somophylin Oral Liquid 2.5 mg/lb/dose po
   Label: Somophylin (aminophylline) Oral Liquid 90 mg/tsp
   Weight: 18 kg
   How many mL should the child receive per dose?

6. **Order:** Omnipen Oral Suspension 50 mg/kg/day in four divided doses
   po
   Label: Omnipen (ampicillin) Oral Suspension 125 mg/5 mL
   Weight: 33 lb
   How many mL should be administered per dose?

7. **Order:** Velosef Expectorant 25 mg/kg in two divided doses po
   Label: Velosef (cephradine) Expectorant 250 mg/5 mL
   Weight: 44 lb
   How many mL should be administered per dose?

8. **Order:** Tetracycline Syrup 25 mg/kg/day in four divided doses po
   Label: Tetracycline Syrup 125 mg/5 mL
   Weight: 37 kg
   How many mL should be administered per dose?

9. **Order:** Amcill Pediatric Drops 50 mg/kg/day in four divided doses po
   Label: Amcill (ampicillin) Pediatric Drops 125 mg/5 mL
   Weight: 42 lb
   How many mL should be administered per dose?

10. **Order:** Antiminth Oral Suspension 5 mg/lb single dose po
    Label: Antiminth (pyrantil pamoate) Oral Suspension 50 mg/mL
    Weight: 45 lb
    How many mL should be administered per dose?

11. **Order:** Cleocin Pediatric 8 mg/kg/day in four divided doses po
    Label: Cleocin (clindamycin) Pediatric 75 mg/5 mL
    Weight: 84 lb
    How many mL should be administered per dose?

12. **Order:** Elixophyllin Elixir 0.3 mL/lb/dose po
    Label: Elixophyllin (theophylline) Elixir 80 mg/15 mL
    Weight: 44 lb
    How many mL should be administered per dose?

13. **Order:** Furadantin Oral Suspension 5 mg/kg in four divided doses po
    Label: Furadantin (nitrofurantoin) Oral Suspension 25 mg/5 mL
    Weight: 15 lb
    How many mL should be administered per dose?

14. **Order:** Pentids 56 mg/kg/day in six divided doses po
    Label: Pentids (penicillin G potassium) Oral Suspension 125 mg/5 mL
    Weight: 38 lb
    How many mL should be administered per dose?

15. **Order:** Penbritin Pediatric Drops Oral Suspension 5 mg/lb/dose po
    Label: Penbritin (ampicillin) Pediatric Drops Oral Suspension 100 mg/mL
    Weight: 12 lb
    How many mL should be administered per dose?

(**Note:** See Appendix G for answer key.)

Calculating Pediatric Dosage—Injections

EXAMPLE

Order: Bicillin LA 50,000 U/kg/day IM in four divided doses

Label: Bicillin LA (Penicillin G Benzathine) 300,000 U/mL

Weight: 50 lb

How many mL will be administered per dose?

Equivalents: 1 kg = 2.2 lb, Bicillin LA 300,000 U = 1 mL, 50,000 U = 1 kg

Conversion Equation:

$$50\;\cancel{lb} \times \frac{1\;\cancel{kg}}{2.2\;\cancel{lb}} \times \frac{50,000\;\cancel{U}}{1\;\cancel{kg}} \times \frac{1\;mL}{300,000\;\cancel{U}}$$

$$= \frac{3.78\;mL}{4\;doses} = 0.95\;mL = 1\;mL$$

(**Note:** When the resulting dosage is less than 1 mL, the answer may be carried to three decimal places and rounded to the nearest hundredth, and the medication may be measured and administered in a tuberculin syringe. If the dosage is 1 mL or more, carry the answer to two decimal places and round to the nearest tenth.)

PRACTICE

Calculating Pediatric Dosage—Injections (see note above)

1. **Order:** Kanamycin Sulfate Injection 15 mg/kg/in two divided doses/day IM
   Label: Figure 12-5. What is the trade name? _____
   Weight: 5 kg
   How many mL should the child receive per dose?

FIGURE 12-5

2. **Order:** Lasix 3 mg/kg IM
   Label: Figure 12-6. What is the generic name? _____
   Weight: 25 lb
   How many mL should the child receive?

FIGURE 12-6

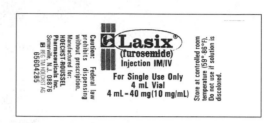

3. **Order:** Keflin 100 mg/kg/day in four divided doses IM
   Label: Keflin (cephalothin) 500 mg/2.2 mL
   Weight: 15 lb
   How many mL should the child receive per dose?

4. **Order:** Streptomycin 30 mg/kg/day in two divided doses IM
   Label: Streptomycin 1 g/2 mL
   Weight: 20 lb
   How many mL should the child receive per dose?

5. **Order:** Polycillin-N 150 mg/kg/day in six divided doses IM
   Label: Polycillin-N (ampicillin) 250 mg/mL
   Weight 55 lb
   How many mL should the child receive per dose?

6. **Order:** Apresoline 1.7 mg/kg/day in four divided doses IM
   Label: Apresoline (hydralazine HCl) 20 mg/mL
   Weight: 12 lb
   How many mL should the child receive per dose?

7. **Order:** Humatrope 0.06 mg/kg/day IM
   Label: Humatrope (somatropin) 5 mg/4 mL
   Weight: 12.2 kg
   How many mL should the child receive per dose?

8. **Order:** Penicillin G Potassium 35,000 U/kg/day in four divided doses IM
   Label: Penicillin G Potassium 250,000 U/mL
   Weight: 72 lb
   How many mL should the child receive per dose?

9. **Order:** Rocephin 50 mg/kg/day in two divided doses IM
   Label: Rocephin (cetriaxone) 250 mg/mL
   Weight: 22.7 kg
   How many mL should the child receive per dose?

10. **Order:** Digoxin 0.002 mg/kg/day in two divided doses IM
    Label: Digoxin 0.5 mg/2 mL
    Weight: 25 lb
    How many mL should the child receive per dose?

(**Note:** See Appendix G for answer key.)

Calculating Pediatric Dosage—IVs

EXAMPLE

Order: Dopamine 5 mcg/kg/min IV. Dilute 100 mg Dopamine in 100 mL D5½NS

Label: Figure 12-7

Weight: 10 lb

FIGURE 12-7

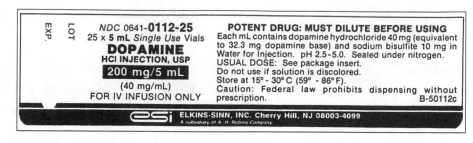

a. How many mL of Dopamine should be added to the 100 mL D5½NS to obtain the ordered dilution?

$$100 \text{ mg} \times \frac{5 \text{ mL}}{200 \text{ mg}} = 2.5 \text{ mL}$$

b. How many mcg of Dopamine should the child receive per min?

$$10 \text{ lb} \times \frac{1 \text{ kg}}{2.2 \text{ lb}} \times \frac{5 \text{ mcg/min}}{1 \text{ kg}} = 22.7 \text{ mcg/min}$$

c. How many mcg of Dopamine should the child receive per hr?

$$1 \text{ hr} \times \frac{60 \text{ min}}{1 \text{ hr}} \times \frac{22.7 \text{ mcg}}{1 \text{ min}} = 1362 \text{ mcg}$$

d. What should the flow rate be in mL/hr to infuse the calculated dose?

$$1 \text{ hr} \times \frac{1362 \text{ mcg}}{1 \text{ hr}} \times \frac{1 \text{ mg}}{1000 \text{ mcg}} \times \frac{100 \text{ mL}}{100 \text{ mg}} = 1 \text{ mL}$$

OR

$$1 \text{ hr} \times \frac{60 \text{ min}}{1 \text{ hr}} \times \frac{22.7 \text{ mcg}}{1 \text{ min}} \times \frac{1 \text{ mg}}{1000 \text{ mcg}} \times \frac{100 \text{ mL}}{100 \text{ mg}} = 1 \text{ mL}$$

e. The infusion pump would be set at an automatic flow rate of 1 mL/hr. Assuming that a microdrip infusion set is being used, what would be the gtt/hr? <u>60</u>

PRACTICE
Calculating Pediatric Dosage—IVs

1. **Order:** Lidocaine 30 mcg/kg/min IV. Dilute 300 mg Lidocaine in 250 mL D5W
   Label: Lidocaine 1 g/25 mL
   Weight: 32.6 kg

   a. How many mL of Lidocaine should be added to the 250 mL D5W to obtain the ordered dilution?

   b. How many mcg of Lidocaine should the child receive per min?

   c. How many mg of Lidocaine should the child receive per hr?

   d. What should the flow rate be in mL/hr to infuse the calculated dose?

   e. At the calculated rate, how many hours should it take for the total IV to infuse?

2. **Order:** Nitropress 2 mcg/kg/min IV. Dilute 30 mg in 250 mL D5½NS
   Label: Nitropress (nitroprusside sodium) 50 mg/2 mL
   Weight: 18.5 kg

   a. How many mL of Nitropress should be added to the 250 mg D5½NS to obtain the ordered dilution?

b. How many mcg of Nitropress should the child receive per min?

c. How many mg of Nitropress should the child receive per hr?

d. What should the flow rate be in mL/hr to infuse the calculated dose?

3. **Order:** Aminophylline 0.3 mg/kg in 30 mL D5W IV to infuse over 20 min
Label: Figure 12-8
Weight: 45 lb

a. How many mg should the child receive as a total dose?

b. How many mL of Aminophylline should be added to the 30 mL D5W?

FIGURE 12-8

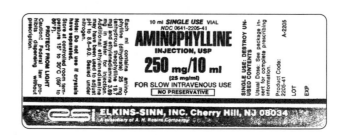

4. **Order:** Verapamil Hydrochloride 0.2 mg/kg via IV bolus
Label: Verapamil Hydrochloride 5 mg/2 mL
Weight: 10 lb
Directions: Administer over a 2 min period.
How much solution should be administered per dose?

5. **Order:** Isoptin 0.3 mg/kg via IV bolus
   Label: Isoptin (verapamil HCl) 5 mg/2 mL
   Weight: 60 lb
   Directions: Administer over a 2 min period.
   How much solution should be administered per dose?

6. **Order:** Monistat IV 20 mg/kg. Administer IV in three divided doses
   Label: Monistat IV (miconazole) 200 mg/20 mL
   Weight: 40 lb
   Directions: Dilute in 200 mL Sodium Chloride 0.9%. Infuse each
   dose in 60 minutes.
   Drop Factor: 60 gtt/mL

   a. How many mL of Monistat IV will contain the ordered dose?

   b. What should the flow rate be?

7. **Order:** Tagamet 5 mg/kg IV in 100 mL D5W. Infuse in 20 min
   Label: Tagamet (cimetidine) 300 mg/2 mL
   Weight: 50 lb
   Drop Factor: 60 gtt/mL

   a. How much Tagamet should be added to the 100 mL D5W?

   b. What should the flow rate be?

8. **Order:** Cosmegen 0.015 mg/kg IV in 50 mL D5W. Administer in 15 min
   Label: Cosmegen (dactinomycin) 0.5 mg/mL
   Weight: 64 lb
   Drop Factor: 60 gtt/mL

   a. How much Cosmegen should be added to the 50 mL D5W?

   b. What should the flow rate be?

(**Note:** See Appendix G for answer key.)

Calculation of Pediatric Dosage Based on Body Surface Area

Pediatric dosage can be calculated on the basis of the body surface area of the child, which can be determined by the use of a nomogram, Figure 12-9. This method can be used for children up to 12 years of age. The child's weight and height are located on the chart; a straight line drawn between them intersects the body-surface column (SA) at the number indicating the child's body surface area (BSA). The surface area measurement is expressed in square meters (M^2). This figure is then plugged into a modified dimensional analysis equation, Figure 12-10, to calculate pediatric dosage using BSA estimates.

The child's body surface area in M^2 is located on the nomogram (Figure 12-9) in the following manner:

Child's height: 26 in

Child's weight: 22 lb

Place a ruler at the level of the child's weight (22 lb) in the right-hand column and line the edge up with the child's height (26 in) in the left-hand column. Read the surface area (SA) measurement at the point where the ruler intersects the SA column. The body surface area for this child is 0.45 M^2.

The enclosed (center) column on the nomogram can be used as an estimate of body surface of children of average height and/or build using weight alone.

FIGURE 12-9 West Nomogram (Modified and reprinted with permission from Begrman, R.E., Kliegman, R.M., and Arvin, A.M. Nelson *Textbook of Pediatrics*, 15th ed., W.B. Saunders Company, Philadelphia, PA 19105)

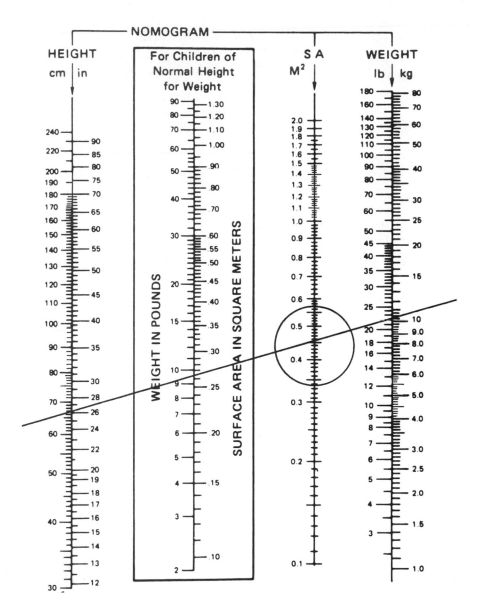

PRACTICE
Use the Nomogram to Determine the Child's Body Surface Area

1. Child's height: 149 cm
   Child's weight: 36 kg
   Body surface area: _____

2. Child's height: 46 in
   Child's weight: 44 lb
   Body surface area: _____

3. Child's height: 138 cm
   Child's weight: 32 kg
   Body surface area: _____

4. Child's height: 29 in
   Child's weight: 22 lb
   Body surface area: _____

5. Child's height: 82 cm
   Child's weight: 12 kg
   Body surface area: _____

(**Note:** See Appendix G for answer key.)

Application of Dimensional Analysis Using BSA Estimates

From the BSA dimensional analysis conversion equation, Figure 12-10, it can be seen that the equivalent relationship between *average adult body surface area* (1.7 M²) and *adult dose* becomes a conversion factor or bridge whereby the *child's BSA* (M²) and the *child's dose* also become an equivalent relationship.

FIGURE 12-10 BSA dimensional analysis conversion equation

$$\text{Child's BSA (M}^2) \times \frac{\text{Adult Dose}}{1.7 \text{ M}^2} = \underline{\hspace{1cm}} \text{ (Child's Dose)}$$

EXAMPLE

Find the child's dose of Amoxicillin

Adult dose: Amoxicillin 250 mg

Child's height: 104 cm
Child's weight: 9.6 kg   From Nomogram: BSA = 0.51 M²

Starting Factor	Answer Unit
Child's BSA (M²)	Child's dose in mg
0.51 M²	_____ mg

Equivalent: 1.7 M² = 250 mg

Conversion Equation: $0.51 \text{ M}^2 \times \dfrac{250 \text{ mg}}{1.7 \text{ M}^2} = 75 \text{ mg}$

PRACTICE

Use Nomogram (Figure 12-9) and Dimensional Analysis to Calculate Pediatric Dosages

(**Note:** Carry to two decimal places and round to nearest tenth.)

1. Child's height: 25 in
   Child's weight: 14 lb
   Adult dose: Meperidine 50 mg
   Find the child's dose.

2. Child's height: 108 cm
   Child's weight: 18 kg
   Adult dose: Mellaril (thioridazine) 10 mg
   Find the child's dose.

3. Child's height: 46 in
   Child's weight: 50 lb
   Adult dose: Xylocaine Hydrochloride 200 mg
   Find the child's dose.

4. Child's height: 54 in
   Child's weight: 70 lb
   Adult dose: Ceftin (cefuroxime) 250 mg
   Find the child's dose.

5. Child's height: 150 cm
   Child's weight: 38 kg
   Adult dose: Augmentin (amoxicillin and potassium clavunate)
   250 mg
   Find the child's dose.

(**Note:** See Appendix G for answer key.)

CHAPTER 13

Clinical Calculations

OBJECTIVE

Upon completion of this chapter you should be able to:

■ Apply dimensional analysis to solve, with 100% accuracy, any type of clinical calculation involved in the administration of medication.

The following clinical problems represent the type of calculations that commonly are encountered in the administration of medications. The prescription orders, the label information, and the conversions required are truly representative of clinical practice. Successful completion of these problems would indicate acceptable competence in performing clinical calculations. With the mastery of this systematic, unified method of problem solving, the learner also should have developed a measure of confidence in his/her ability to solve new problems as they may occur in the clinical setting.

Although most of the equivalent relationships should have been memorized by now, it may be helpful to detach the table of equivalents (printed on the back of title page) for use as a reference in completing the following calculations and for future use in the clinical area.

Before beginning this unit, you may wish to review the method (and modifications) for determining the starting factor and answer unit.

■ In general, the starting factor is the known quantity and its unit which is to be converted to a desired unit (quantity of medication).

EXAMPLE   Starting Factor   Answer Unit
                  gr, g   mg, cap, tsp

■ In calculations based on body weight, the starting factor is the particular quantity of weight that is to be converted to a desired unit (quantity of medication).

EXAMPLE   Starting Factor   Answer Unit
                  lb, kg   mL, mg, tab ÷ number of doses

■ In calculations based on body surface area, the starting factor is the particular amount of body surface area that is to be converted to a desired unit (child's dose).

EXAMPLE   Starting Factor   Answer Unit
                  BSA (M^2)   mg, mL, gtt

■ In calculations for IV flow rate in gtt/min, the starting factor is the particular amount of time (1 min) that is to be converted to a desired unit (number of drops).

EXAMPLE   Starting Factor   Answer Unit
                    min   gtt

- In calculations for IV flow rate in mL/hr, the starting factor is the particular amount of time (1 hr) that is to be converted to a desired unit (number of mL).

EXAMPLE   Starting Factor   Answer Unit
                    hr   mL

- In calculations for IV infusion time, the starting factor is the particular amount of solution (mL) that is to be converted to a desired unit (amount of time).

EXAMPLE   Starting Factor   Answer Unit
                    mL   hr, min, sec

PRACTICE
Solve Using Dimensional Analysis

(**Note:** Round in the appropriate manner. Assume that parenteral dosages of less than 1 mL will be administered via tuberculin syringe.)

1. **Order:** Restoril gr $\overline{ss}$ po
   Label: Figure 13-1

FIGURE 13-1

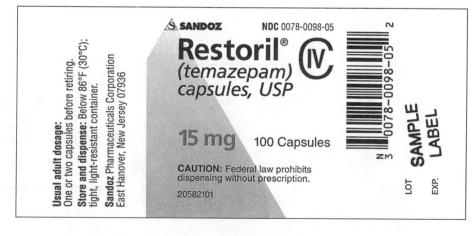

2. **Order:** Colchicine gr 1/200 po
   Label: Colchicine 0.6 mg/tab (scored)

3. **Order:** Lanoxin 0.125 mg po
   Label: Lanoxin (digoxin) 0.25 mg/tab (scored)

4. **Order:** Dynapen Oral Suspension 125 mg po
   Label: Dynapen (dicloxacillin sodium) Oral Suspension 62.5 mg/
   5 mL

5. **Order:** Prostaphlin 0.5 g po
   Label: Prostaphlin (oxacillin sodium) 250 mg/cap

6. **Order:** Dramamine 100 mg po
   Label: Dramamine (dimenhydrinate) 50 mg/tab

7. **Order:** Keflex 0.5 g po
   Label: Figure 13-2

FIGURE 13-2

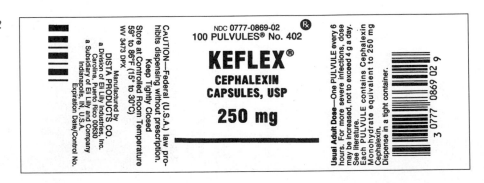

8. **Order:** Zyloprim 0.3 g po
   Label: Zyloprim (allopurinol) 100 mg/tab

9. **Order:** Vibramycin Syrup 125 mg po
   Label: Vibramycin (doxycycline calcium oral suspension) Syrup 50 mg/tsp
   Give _____ mL

10. **Order:** Codeine Sulfate gr/po
    Label: Figure 13-3

FIGURE 13-3

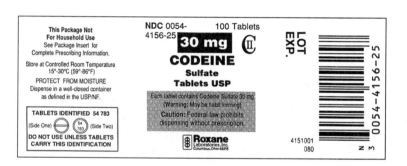

11. **Order:** V Cillin K Oral Suspension 125 mg po
    Label: V Cillin K (penicillin V potassium) Oral Suspension 250 mg/ 5 mL

12. **Order:** Chloral Hydrate Suspension 0.75 g po
    Label: Chloral Hydrate Suspension 0.5 g/ʒ 1
    Give _____ mL

13. **Order:** Dalmane Cap 30 mg po
    Label: Figure 13-4

FIGURE 13-4

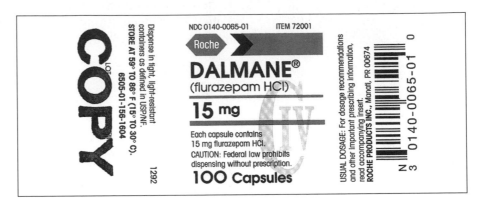

14. **Order:** Mysoline Suspension 125 mg po
    Label: Mysoline (primidone) Suspension 0.25 g/5 mL

15. **Order:** Vistaril Oral Suspension 50 mg po
    Label: Figure 13-5
    Give _____ tsp

FIGURE 13-5

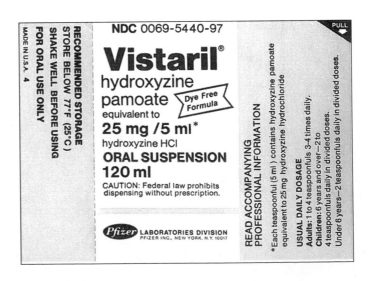

16. **Order:** Riopan 10 mL po
    Label: Riopan (magaldrate) 400 mg/tsp
    Give _____ mg

17. **Order:** Saluron 0.15 g po
    Label: Saluron (hydroflumethiazide) 50 mg/tab

18. **Order:** Klorvess 30 mEq po
    Label: Klorvess (potassium chloride) 20 mEq/15 mL

19. **Order:** Nitrostat gr $\frac{1}{400}$ sl
    Label: Figure 13-6

FIGURE 13-6

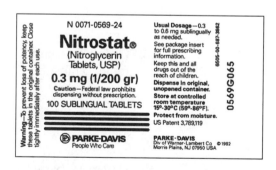

20. **Order:** Gantrisin gr 8 po
    Label: Gantrisin (sulfasoxazole) 250 mg/tab

21. **Order:** Actidil 0.6 mg po
    Label: Actidil (triprolidine) 1.25 mg/5 mL

22. **Order:** Phenobarbital gr s̅s̅ po
    Label: Figure 13-7

FIGURE 13-7

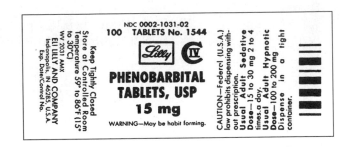

23. **Order:** Polycillin Oral Suspension gr viis̅s̅ po
    Label: Polycillin (ampicillin) Oral Suspension 125 mg/5 mL

24. **Order:** Premarin 1.25 mg po
    Label: Premarin (estrogens conjugated) 0.625 mg/tab

25. **Order:** Thiosulfil Forte 0.25 g po
    Label: Thiosulfil Forte (sulfamethizole) 500 mg/tab (scored)

26. **Order:** Mebaral 0.64 g po
    Label: Mebaral (mephobarbital) 320 mg/tab

27. **Order:** Paradione Capsules 0.9 g po
    Label: Paradione (paramethadione) 300 mg/cap

28. **Order:** Ceclor Cap 500 mg po
    Label: Figure 13-8

FIGURE 13-8

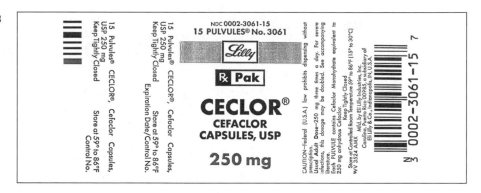

29. **Order:** Crystodigin 0.15 mg po
    Label: Crystodigin (digitoxin) 0.1 mg/tab (scored)

30. **Order:** Quinora 0.6 g po
    Label: Quinora (quinidine sulfate) gr iii/tab

31. **Order:** Slow-K tab 2400 mg po
    Label: Figure 13-9

FIGURE 13-9

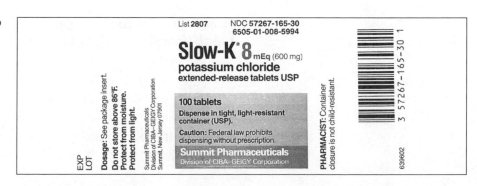

32. **Order:** Isosorbide dinetrate 80 mg po
    Label: Figure 13-10

FIGURE 13-10

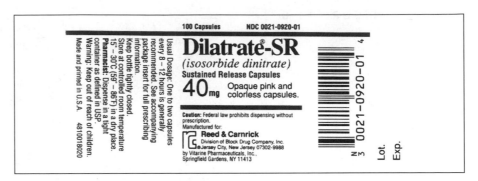

33. **Order:** Tylenol gr v po
    Label: Tylenol (acetaminophen) 325 mg/tab

34. **Order:** Pen-Vee K 250 mg po
    Label: Pen-Vee K (penicillin V potassium) 125 mg/tsp
    Give _____ mL

35. **Order:** Mellaril 75 mg po
    Label: Mellaril (thioridazine) 30 mg/mL

36. **Order:** Choledyl Elixir 0.2 g po
    Label: Choledyl (oxtriphylline) Elixir 100 mg/5 mL

37. **Order:** Caffeine gr iii po
    Label: Caffeine 0.2 g/tab

38. **Order:** Librium Cap 10 mg po
    Label: Figure 13-11

FIGURE 13-11

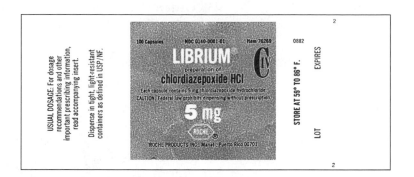

39. **Order:** Halcion 0.125 mg po
    Label: Figure 13-12

FIGURE 13-12

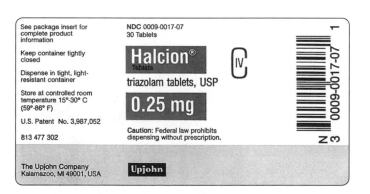

40. **Order:** Aldomet 500 mg po
    Label: Aldomet (methyldopa) 125 mg/tab

41. **Order:** Phenergan 25 mg po
    Label: Phenergan (promethazine HCl) 12.5 mg/tab

42. **Order:** Erythromycin 0.75 g po
    Label: Erythromycin 250 mg/cap

43. **Order:** Hydroxzine pamoate oral suspension 60 mg po
    Label: Figure 13-13

FIGURE 13-13

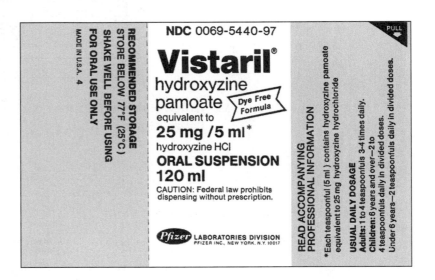

44. **Order:** Quinidine Sulfate gr 6 po
    Label: Quinidine Sulfate 0.2 g/tab

45. **Order:** Gantrisin 2 g po
    Label: Gantrisin (sulfasoxizole) 500 mg/tab

46. **Order:** Nitroglycerin gr $\frac{1}{600}$ sublingual
    Label: Nitroglycerin 0.1 mg/tab

47. **Order:** Carbamazepine tab 0.2 g po
    Label: Figure 13-14

FIGURE 13-14

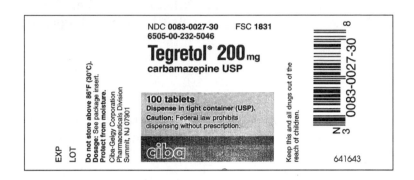

48. **Order:** Chloral Hydrate Elixir 1.0 g po
    Label: Chloral Hydrate Elixir gr viiss̄/5 mL

49. **Order:** Penicillin V Potassium oral Sol. 100,000 U po
    Label: Figure 13-15

FIGURE 13-15

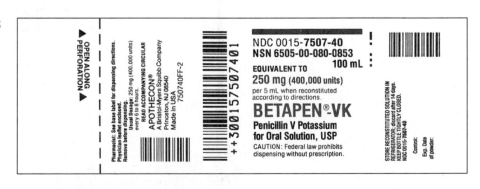

50. **Order:** Naloxone HCl 0.4 mg IM
    Label: Naloxone HCl 400 mcg (μg)/mL

51. **Order:** Pfizerpen AS 500,000 U IM
    Label: Pfizerpen AS (penicillin G procaine) 300,000 U/mL

52. **Order:** Librium 25 mg IM
    Label: Librium (chlordiazepoxide) 100 mg/2 mL

53. **Order:** Terramycin 100 mg IM
    Label: Terramycin (oxytetracycline) 250 mg/2 mL

54. **Order:** Nebcin 55 mg IM
    Label: Figure 13-16

FIGURE 13-16

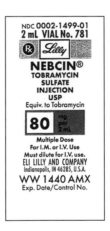

55. **Order:** Meperidine 60 mg IM
    Label: Meperidine 75 mg/1.5 mL

56. Order: Ergotrate 0.15 mg IM
Label: Ergotrate (ergonovine maleate) 0.2 mg/mL

57. Order: Vitamin B₁₂ 600 mcg IM
Label: Vitamin B₁₂ (cyanocobalamin) 1000 mcg/mL

58. Order: Lanoxin 0.25 mg IM
Label: Figure 13-17

FIGURE 13-17

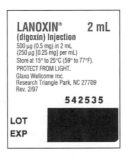

59. Order: Kantrex 500 mg IM
Label: Kantrex (kanamycin sulfate) 1 g/3 mL

60. Order: Kanamycin Sulfate 10 mg IM
Label: Kanamycin Sulfate 75 mg/2 mL

61. Order: Vistaril 25 mg IM
Label: Vistaril (hydroxyzine HCl) 100 mg/2 mL

62. **Order:** Digitoxin 0.05 mg IM
    Label: Digitoxin 0.2 mg/2 mL

63. **Order:** Promethazine gr ⅙ IM
    Label: Promethazine 25 mg/mL

64. **Order:** Cefadyl 0.75 g IM
    Label: Figure 13-18

FIGURE 13-18

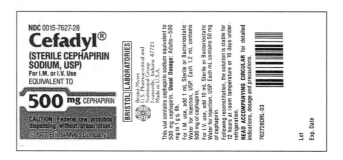

65. **Order:** Lasix 40 mg IM
    Label: Lasix (furosemide) 10 mg/mL

66. **Order:** Thorazine 15 mg IM
    Label: Thorazine (chlorpromazine) 25 mg/mL

67. **Order:** Atropine Sulfate gr ¹⁄₁₅₀ sc
    Label: Atropine Sulfate gr ¹⁄₁₀₀ per mL

68. **Order:** Ancef 250 mg IM
    Label: Figure 13-19

FIGURE 13-19   *(Courtesy
SmithKline Beecham
Pharmaceuticals)*

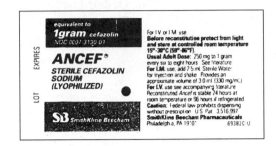

69. **Order:** Tetracyn 100 mg IM
    Label: Tetracyn (tetracycline HCl) 250 mg/1.8 mL

70. **Order:** Meperidine 15 mg IM
    Label: Meperidine 25 mg/mL

71. **Order:** Achromycin 0.2 g IM
    Label: Achromycin (tetracycline HCl) 250 mg/2 mL

72. **Order:** Thorazine 12.5 mg IM
    Label: Figure 13-20

FIGURE 13-20

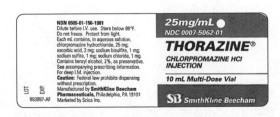

73. **Order:** Serpasil 2.5 mg IM
  Label: Serpasil (reserpine) 5 mg/mL

74. **Order:** Phenergan 35 mg IM
  Label: Figure 13-21

FIGURE 13-21

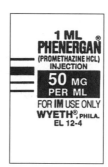

75. **Order:** Kantrex 1000 mg IM
  Label: Kantrex (kanamycin sulfate) 0.5 g/2 mL

76. **Order:** Polycillin 0.125 g IM
  Label: Polycillin (ampicillin) 250 mg/1.5 mL

77. **Order:** Demerol 30 mg IM
  Label: Figure 13-22

FIGURE 13-22

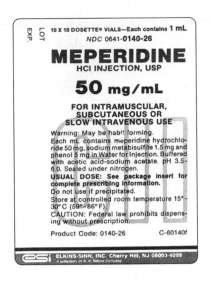

78. **Order:** Morphine Sulfate gr $\frac{1}{12}$ sc
    Label: Morphine Sulfate 10 mg/mL

79. **Order:** Atropine Sulfate gr $\frac{1}{150}$ IM
    Label: Figure 13-23

FIGURE 13-23

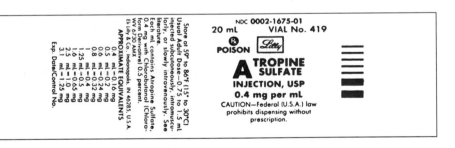

80. **Order:** Morphine Sulfate 10 mg IM
    Label: Figure 13-24

FIGURE 13-24

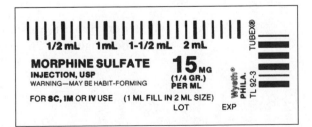

81. **Order:** Tagamet 200 mg IM
    Label: Tagamet (cimetidine) 300 mg/2 mL in prefilled syringe
    Give _____ mL
    Discard _____ mL

82. **Order:** Terramycin 150 mg IM
    Label: Terramycin (oxytetracycline) 50 mg/mL

83. **Order:** Zantac 15 mg IM
    Label: Figure 13-25

FIGURE 13-25

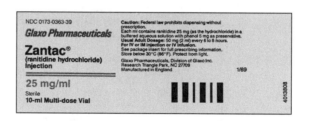

84. **Order:** Nembutal 60 mg IM
    Label: Nembutal (pentobarbital) 100 mg/2 mL

85. **Order:** Kanamycin Sulfate 750 mg IM
    Label: Kanamycin Sulfate 1 g/3 mL

86. **Order:** Heparin Sodium 7000 U sc
    Label: Figure 13-26

FIGURE 13-26

NDC 0009-0317-02
4 ml

**Heparin Sodium
Injection, USP**
Sterile Solution

10,000 Units per ml
from beef lung

For subcutaneous o.
intravenous use

See package insert for complete
product information.

Store at controlled room temperature
15°-30° C (59°-86° F).

Each ml contains: Heparin sodium,
10,000 USP units.

811 331 201

The Upjohn Company
Kalamazoo, MI 49001, USA

87. **Order:** Valium 8 mg IM
   Label: Valium (diazepam) 0.1 g/2 mL

88. **Order:** Atropine Sulfate 0.3 mg IM
   Label: Atropine Sulfate 0.4 mg/mL

89. **Order:** Vitamin B_{12} 750 mcg IM
   Label: Vitamin B_{12} 1000 mcg/mL

90. **Order:** Ceftazidime 0.25 g IM
   Label: Figure 13-27

FIGURE 13-27

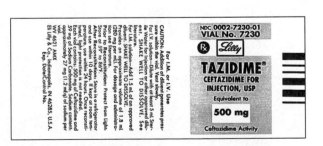

91. **Order:** Aqua Mephyton 0.5 mg IM
   Label: Aqua Mephyton (phytonadione) 2 mg/mL

92. **Order:** Methicillin Sodium 750 mg IM
    Label: Methicillin Sodium 1 g dry powder
    Reconstitution: Add 1.5 mL sterile water for injection to yield 0.5 g/mL.

93. **Order:** Streptomycin 400 mg IM
    Label: Streptomycin 1 g dry powder
    Reconstitution: Add 3.2 mL sterile water for injection to yield 250 mg/mL.

94. **Order:** Ampicillin 350 mg IM
    Label: Ampicillin 2 g dry powder
    Reconstitution: Add 6.8 mL sterile water for injection to yield 250 mg/mL.

95. **Order:** Potassium Penicillin G 40,000 U IM
    Label: Potassium Penicillin G 400,000 U dry powder
    Reconstitution: Add 4 mL sterile saline for injection to yield 100,000 U/mL.

96. **Order:** Ampicillin 500 mg IM
    Label: Ampicillin 1 g dry powder
    Reconstitution: Add 2.4 mL sterile water for injection to yield 1 g/2.5 mL.

97. **Order:** Ticar 650 mg IM
    Label: Figure 13-28

FIGURE 13-28

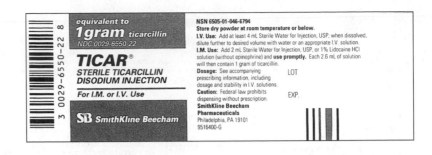

98. Order: Polymyxin B 50 mg IM
Label: Polymyxin B 150 mg dry powder
Reconstitution: Add 2 mL sterile diluent to yield 0.075 g/mL.

99. Order: Penicillin G Potassium 750 mg IM
Label: Penicillin G Potassium 5 g dry powder
Reconstitution: Add 9.6 mL sterile diluent to yield 1 g/2.2 mL.

100. Order: Keflex 500 mg IM
Label: Keflex 5 g dry powder (cephalexin) 5 g dry powder
Reconstitution: Add 10 mL sterile diluent to yield 0.5 g/mL.

101. Order: Kefzol 250 mg IM
Label: Figure 13-29

FIGURE 13-29

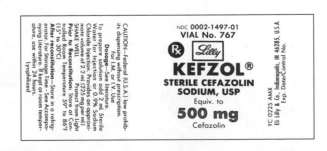

102. **Order:** Moxalactam Disodium 300 mg IM
Label: Figure 13-30

FIGURE 13-30

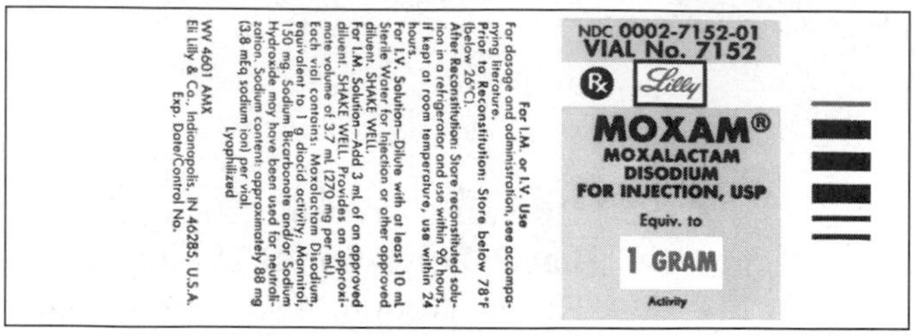

103. **Order:** Mezlin 0.6 g IM
Label: Mezlin (mezlocillin) 1 g dry powder
Reconstitution: Add 4 mL sterile water for injection to yield 250 mg/mL.

104. **Order:** Pipracil 1200 mg IM
Label: Pipracil (piperacillin) 2 g dry powder
Reconstitution: For each gram, add 2 mL of sterile diluent to yield 1 g/2.5 mL.

105. **Order:** Ampicillin 150 mg IM
Label: Ampicillin 1 g dry powder
Reconstitution: Add 3.4 mL sterile water for injection to yield 1 g/4 mL.

106. **Order:** Cefazolin Sodium 500 mg IM
Label: Cefazolin Sodium 1 g dry powder
Reconstitution: Add 3 mL sterile water for injection to yield 1 g/3 mL.

107. **Order:** Ritalin 5 mg IM
     Label: Ritalin (methylphenidate HCl) 100 mg dry powder
     Reconstitution: Add 10 mL sterile aqueous solvent to yield 100 mg/10 mL.

108. **Order:** BCG vaccine 400,000 U ID
     Label: BCG vaccine 8,000,000 U/mL

109. **Order:** Vitamin A 17,500 U IM
     Label: Vitamin A 50,000 U/mL

110. **Order:** Vitamin A 35,000 U IM
     Label: Vitamin A 50,000 U/mL

For 111–160, calculate flow rate in gtt/min unless directed otherwise.

111. **Order:** 3000 mL D5W IV in 24 hr
     Drop Factor: 15 gtt/mL

112. **Order:** 750 mL 5% D5NS IV in 6 hr
     Drop Factor: 15 gtt/mL

113. **Order:** 2500 mL Lactated Ringers IV in 24 hr
     Drop Factor: 15 gtt/mL

114. **Order:** 1000 mL D5W IV in 4 hr
Drop Factor: 10 gtt/mL

115. **Order:** 1.5 L NS IV in 8 hr
Drop Factor: 20 gtt/mL

116. **Order:** 1000 mL Ringers Solution IV in 8 hr
Drop Factor: 15 gtt/mL

117. **Order:** 250 mL packed blood cells IV in 4 hr
Drop Factor: 10 gtt/mL

118. **Order:** 650 mL D5W in 3 hr, IV
Drop Factor: 10 gtt/mL

119. **Order:** 1000 mL Ringers Solution IV in 8 hr
Drop Factor: 10 gtt/mL

120. **Order:** 300 mL 10% Glucose in 8 hr, IV
Drop Factor: 10 gtt/mL

121. **Order:** 100 mL 10% Glucose in 3 hr, IV
Drop Factor: 15 gtt/mL

122. **Order:** 2000 mL D5W in 12 hr, IV
     Drop Factor: 10 gtt/mL

123. **Order:** 500 mL D5W in 4 hr, IV
     Drop Factor: 10 gtt/mL

124. **Order:** 1200 mL D5W in 8 hr, IV
     Drop Factor: 15 gtt/mL

125. **Order:** 900 mL NS in 6 hr, IV
     Drop Factor: 10 gtt/mL

126. **Order:** 500 mL D5W in 3.5 hr, IV
     Drop Factor: 15 gtt/mL

127. **Order:** 2000 mL of D5W in 24 hr, IV
     Drop Factor: 10 gtt/mL

128. **Order:** 500 mL Normal Saline in 12 hr, IV
     Drop Factor: 60 gtt/mL

129. **Order:** 3000 mL D5W in 24 hr, IV
     Drop Factor: 15 gtt/mL

130. **Order:** 1000 mL Lactated Ringers in 12 hr, IV
     Drop Factor: 60 gtt/mL

131. **Order:** 750 mL Ringers Solution in 5 hr, IV
     Drop Factor: 10 gtt/mL

132. **Order:** Areosporin 50 mg in 250 mL sterile water IV in 1 ½ hr
     Drop Factor: 15 gtt/mL

133. **Order:** Neosporin (bacitracin) GU Irrigant 1 amp in 1000 cc Isotonic
     Saline IV in 24 hr
     Drop Factor: 10 gtt/mL

134. **Order:** Staphcillin (methicillin sodium) 500 mg in 50 mL NS IV at 10
     mL/min
     Drop Factor: 15 gtt/mL

135. **Order:** Monistat IV 200 mg diluted in 200 mL NS IV in 2 hr
     Label: Monistat IV (miconazole) 200 mg/20 mL
     Drop Factor: 60 gtt/mL

     a. How many mL of Monistat IV should be added to the 200 mL
        NS?

     b. What should the flow rate be? (Omit 5% rule.)

136. **Order:** Penicillin G Potassium 15,000,000 U IV in 1000 mL D5W to infuse over 24 hr
Label: Penicillin G Potassium 20,000,000 U
Reconstitution: Dilute with 31.6 mL of D5W to yield 500,000 U/mL.
Drop Factor: 15 gtt/mL

 a. How much should be added to the 1000 mL of D5W?

 b. What should the flow rate be? (Use 5% rule.)

137. **Order:** 2500 mL D5W IV
Drop Factor: 10 gtt/mL
Flow Rate: 40 gtt/min
How long should it take the IV to infuse?

138. **Order:** Zovirax 5 mg/kg IVPB in 100 mL D5W in 60 min
Weight: 70 kg
Label: Zovirax (acyclovir) 500 mg dry powder
Drop Factor: 60 gtt/mL
Directions: Reconstitute by adding 10 mL sterile diluent to yield 50 mg/mL.

 a. How many mL of reconstituted Zovirax should be added to the 100 mL D5W?

 b. What should the flow rate be? (Omit 5% rule.)

139. **Order:** Aminophylline 1 g in 1000 mL D5½NS IV to infuse at 35 mg/hr
Drop Factor: 60 gtt/mL
What should the flow rate be?

140. **Order:** Mefoxin 2 g IVPB in 100 mL Sodium Chloride 0.9% in 60 min
    Label: Mefoxin (cefoxitan sodium) 1 g dry powder
    Reconstitution: Dilute with 10 mL sterile water for injection to yield 1 g/10.5 mL.
    Drop Factor: 15 gtt/mL

    a. How many mL Mefoxin should be added to the IV solution?

    b. What should the flow rate be? (Use 5% rule.)

141. **Order:** Cefazolin Sodium 1 g in 100 mL 10% DW IV to infuse in 60 min via Volutrol
    Label: Cefazolin Sodium 1 g dry powder
    Reconstitution: Dilute with 2.5 mL sterile water for injection to yield 1 g/3 mL.
    Drop Factor: 60 gtt/mL
    What should the flow rate be?

142. **Order:** Heparin Sodium 30,000 U in 250 mL D5W IV to infuse at 10 mL/hr (via IV pump)
    Label: Heparin Sodium 20,000 U/mL
    Drop Factor: 60 gtt/mL

    a. How many mL of Heparin should be added to the IV solution?

    b. What should the flow rate be? (Use 5% rule.)

143. **Order:** Heparin Sodium 10,000 U in 100 mL D5W IV to infuse at 1200 U/hr
    Label: Heparin Sodium 10,000 U/mL
    Drop Factor: 60 gtt/mL

    a. What should the flow rate be?

    b. How many hours will it take to complete the IV?

144. Order: Regular Insulin 10 U/hr IV in 500 mL NS to infuse in 6 hr
Label: Regular Insulin 100 U/mL
How many units of Insulin should be added to the IV solution in order to administer the Insulin over a period of 6 hrs?

145. Order: Lidocaine HCl 1 g in 250 mL D5W (IV minibottle/saline lock) to infuse at a rate of 2 mg/min
Label: Lidocaine HCl 1g/5 mL
Drop Factor: 60 gtt/mL
What should the flow rate be?

146. Order: Dopamine HCl 400 mg in 500 mL D5W to infuse at 5 mcg/kg/min IV
Weight: 75 kg
Drop Factor: 60 gtt/mL

    a. How many mcg/min should be administered?

    b. How many mL/hr will provide the required dose?

    c. How many gtt/min will provide the required dose?

    d. How many mcg/gtt will be administered?

147. Order: Heparin Sodium 7000 U in 250 mL D5W at 0.4 U/kg/min IV
Weight: 129 lb
Drop Factor: 60 gtt/mL

    a. How many U/min should be administered?

    b. How many mL/hr will provide the required dose?

    c. How many gtt/min will provide the required dose?

148. Order: Nipride (nitroprusside sodium) 50 mg in 250 mL D5W at 4
mcg/kg/min IV
Weight: 77.6 kg
Drop Factor: 60 gtt/mL

    a. How many mcg/min should be administered?

    b. How many mL/hr will provide the required dose?

    c. How many gtt/min will provide the required dose?

    d. How many mcg/gtt will be administered?

149. **Order:** Dobutamine HCl 250 mg in 500 mL 5% Dextrose in Lactated Ringers at 10 mcg/kg/min IV
Weight: 181 lb
Drop Factor: 60 gtt/mL

   a. How many mcg/min should be administered?

   b. How many mL/hr will provide the required dose?

   c. How many gtt/min will provide the required dose?

   d. How many mcg/gtt will be administered?

150. **Order:** Intropin (dopamine HCl) 400 mg in 500 mL D5W at 10 mcg/kg/min IV
Weight: 88.6 kg
Drop Factor: 60 gtt/mL

   a. How many mcg/min should be administered?

   b. How many mL/hr will provide the required dose?

   c. How many gtt/min will provide the required dose?

   d. How many mcg/gtt will be administered?

151. Order: Nitroprusside Sodium 50 mg in 250 mL D5W at 4
mcg/kg/min IV
Weight: 109 lb
Drop Factor: 60 gtt/mL

  a. How many mcg/min should be administered?

  b. How many mL/hr will provide the required dose?

  c. How many gtt/min will provide the required dose?

  d. How many mcg/gtt will be administered?

152. Order: Infuse Nitroprusside Sodium 50 mg in 250 mL D5W. Titrate
0.5–1.5 mcg/kg/min to maintain the systolic blood pressure below
140 mm Hg.
Weight: 198 lb

  a. What is the concentration of the solution in mcg/mL?

  b. How many mcg/min will administer the ordered range of titration?
Lower (0.5 mcg/kg/min):

  Upper (1.5 mcg/kg/min):

  c. How many mL/hr or gtt/min will administer the ordered range
of titration?

Lower:

Upper:

d. What is the titration (concentration) factor in mcg/gtt?

e. The present systolic blood pressure reading is 155 mm Hg. Increase the gtt/min by 5 gtt. How many mcg/min will the patient now be receiving?

153. Order: Heparin Sodium 25,000 U in 500 mL D5W IV to infuse over 24 hr via IV pump
To how many mL/hr should the IV pump be set?

154. Order: Penicillin G Potassium 8 million units IVPB in 100 mL D5W to infuse over 1 hr
Label: Penicillin G Potassium 20,000,000 U dry powder
Reconstitution: Add 11.5 mL sterile water for injection to yield 1,000,000 U/mL.
Drop Factor: 15 gtt/mL

a. How many mL of reconstituted solution should be added to 100 mL D5W?

b. What should the flow rate be? (Omit 5% rule.)

155. Order: KCl 40 mEq in 1000 mL D5W IV
Drop Factor: 15 gtt/mL
Flow Rate: 35 gtt/min
How long should it take the IV to infuse?

156. Order: Aminophylline 150 mg IVPB in 100 mL D5W to infuse in 60 min
Label: Aminophylline 250 mg/10 mL
Drop Factor: 60 gtt/mL

   a. How many mL should be added to the 100 mL D5W?

   b. What should the flow rate be? (Use 5% rule.)

157. Order: Zovirax (acyclovir) 5 mg/kg IVPB in 100 mL D5W to infuse in 60 min
Label: Zovirax 500 mg dry powder
Weight: 130 lb
Reconstitution: Add 10 mL sterile water for injection to yield 500 mg/10 mL.
Drop Factor: 60 gtt/mL

   a. How many mL should be added to the 100 mL D5W?

   b. What should the flow rate be? (Omit 5% rule.)

158. Order: Achromycin 500 mg IVPB in 100 mL D5W to infuse in 1 hr
Label: Achromycin (tetracycline HCl) 0.5 g dry powder
Reconstitution: Add 10 mL sterile diluent to yield 250 mg per 5 mL.
Drop Factor: 15 gtt/mL

a. How many mL of reconstituted solution should be added to 100 mL D5W?

b. What should the flow rate be? (Use 5% rule.)

159. Order: Vistaril (hydroxyzine HCl) 75 mg in 100 mL NS IV via Metriset
Drop Factor: 60 gtt/mL
Flow Rate: 100 gtt/min
How long should it take the IV to infuse?

160. Order: 1000 mL D5½NS IV via central venous catheter to infuse at 150 mL/hr for first 500 mL. Add MVI 10 mL to remaining 500 mL and continue infusion at 75 mL/hr. Use an IV pump.
Label: MVI 10 mL/ampule
Drop Factor: 60 gtt/mL

a. What should the flow rate be for the first 500 mL?

b. To what should the flow rate be adjusted for the remaining 500 mL?

161. Order: Heparin Sodium 10,000 U in 100 mL D5W IV to infuse at 10 gtt/min
Drop Factor: 60 gtt/mL
How many units of Heparin is the patient receiving in 24 hours?

162. **Order:** Digoxin 0.375 mg IV Push at a rate of 0.5 mL/min
     Label: Digoxin 0.25 mg/mL

     a. How many mL of Digoxin should be administered?

     b. How long should it take to administer the IV Digoxin?

163. **Order:** Lidocaine HCl 1 mg/kg via IV Push
     Weight: 154 lb
     How many mg should be administered per dose?

164. **Order:** Adriamycin 30 mg/M^2 via IV bolus at a rate of 3 mg/min
     BSA = 0.5 M^2
     Label: Adriamycin (doxorubicin HCl) 10 mg. Dilute in 5 mL sodium
     chloride for injection.

     a. How many mL should be administered per dose?

     b. How long should it take to inject the Adriamycin?

165. **Order:** Valium (0.3 mg/kg via IV bolus at a rate of 5 mg/min
     Label: Valium (diazepam) 5 mg/mL
     Weight: 40 lb

     a. How many mL of Valium should the child receive per dose?

     b. How long should it take to inject the Valium?

166. **Order:** Lorfan 0.02 mg/kg of body weight via IV push at a rate of 1 mg/min
   Label: Lorfan (levallorphan tartrate) 0.4 mg/mL
   Weight: 35 lb

   a. How many mL of Lorfan should the child receive per dose?

   b. How long should it take to inject the Lorfan?

167. **Order:** TPN 1000 mL Liposyn II 20% IV
   How many kcal of fat are provided?

168. **Order:** CPN 1000 mL 5% dextrose in 0.9% Sodium Chloride IV
   How many kcal of carbohydrate are provided?

169. **Order:** PTPN 500 mL Aminosyn II 3.5% IV
   How many kcal of protein are provided?

170. **Order:** Hyperalimentation 1500 mL Liposyn 10% IV
   How many kcal of fat are provided?

171. **Order:** Methimazole 0.4 mg/kg po in three divided doses
   Label: Methimazole 5 mg/tab (scored)
   Weight: 79 lb

172. **Order:** Valproic Acid 5 mg/kg po in three divided doses
     Label: Valproic Acid 250 mg/5 mL
     Weight: 165 lb

173. **Order:** Isoniazid 5 mg/kg po
     Label: Isoniazid 100 mg/tab
     Weight: 60 kg

174. **Order:** Sus-Phrine 0.005 mL/kg sc
     Label: Sus-Phrine (epinephrine) 2.5 mg/5 mL
     Weight: 44 lb

175. **Order:** Paromomycin 25 mg/kg/day po in three divided doses
     Label: Paromomycin 250 mg/capsule
     Weight: 160 lb
     How many capsules should be administered/dose?

176. **Order:** Symmetrel Syrup 8.8 mg/kg po in two divided doses
     Label: Symmetrel (amantadine) Syrup 50 mg/5 mL
     Weight: 35 lb

177. **Order:** Terramycin 3 mg/lb/day in two divided doses IM
     Label: Terramycin (oxytetracycline) 100 mg/2 mL
     Weight: 20 lb

178. **Order:** Kantrex 15 mg/kg/day in two divided doses IM
     Label: Kantrex (kanamycin sulfate) 75 mg/2 mL
     Weight: 55 lb

179. Order: Lomotil Liquid 0.4 mg/kg/day in 4 divided doses po
  Label: Figure 13-31
  Weight: 50 lb

FIGURE 13-31

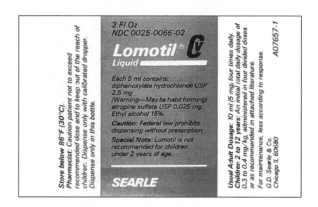

180. Order: Tetracyn Syrup 50 mg/kg/day in four divided doses po
  Label: Tetracyn (tetracycline HCl) Syrup 125 mg/tsp
  Weight: 60 lb
  Give _____ mL/dose

181. Order: Nebcin 7.5 mg/kg/day in 4 divided doses IM
  Label: Figure 13-32
  Weight: 15 kg

FIGURE 13-32

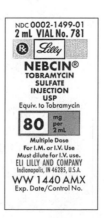

182. **Order:** Dobutrex 250 mg in 500 mL 5% Dextrose IV at 5 mcg
    (μg)/kg/min
    Label: Dobutrex (dobutamine HCl) 250 mg/20 mL
    Weight: 143 lb

183. **Order:** Rondomycin Syrup 6 mg/lb/day in four divided doses po
    Label: Rondomycin (methacycline) Syrup 75 mg/5 mL
    Weight: 62 lb

184. **Order:** Kefzol 25 mg/kg/day in four divided doses IM
    Label: Kefzol (cefazolin sodium) 250 mg dry powder
    Weight: 30 lb
    Reconstitution: Dilute in 2 mL sterile water for injection to yield
    125 mg/mL.

185. **Order:** Acetaminophen Elixir 10 mg/kg/dose po
    Label: Acetaminophen Elixir 160 mg/5 mL
    Weight: 54 lb

For 186–190, use the West nomogram and dimensional analysis.

186. Child's height: 33 in
    Child's weight: 28 lb
    Adult dose: Dilantin (phenytoin sodium) 100 mg
    Find the child's dose.

187. Child's height: 95 cm
    Child's weight: 15 kg
    Adult dose: Lomotil (diphenoxylate HCl and atropine sulfate) 5 mL
    Find the child's dose.

188. Child's height: 104 cm
Child's weight: 17 kg
Adult dose: Atropine Sulfate 0.4 mg
Find the child's dose.

189. Child's height: 52 in
Child's weight: 50 lb
Adult dose: Digoxin 0.125 mg
Find the child's dose.

190. Child's height: 58.5 cm
Child's weight: 5.9 kg
Adult dose: Valium (diazepam) 2 mg
Find the child's dose.

For 191–200, use the drug labels in Figure 13-33 and calculate the correct dosage.

191. Order: Ticar (ticarcillin) 250 mg IM

192. Order: Ilosone Oral Suspension 150 mg po

193. Order: Pitressin 8 Units sc

194. Order: Heparin Sodium 3000 U sc

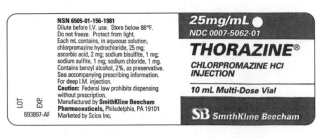

a.

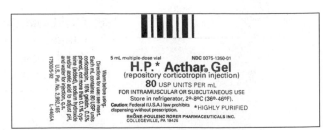

b.

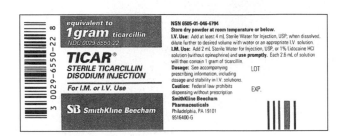

c.

N 0469-2067-15 Sterile. Nonpyrogenic. 967-20

MUST BE DILUTED PRIOR TO IV ADMINISTRATION

LyphoMed®
POTASSIUM CHLORIDE
INJECTION, USP
(2 mEq/mL)

20 mL
Multiple Dose Vial
40 mEq

Each mL contains: Potassium Chloride 149 mg;
Methylparaben 0.05%; Propylparaben 0.005%;
Water for Injection q.s. pH adjusted with HCl or
KOH if necessary. 4000 mOsmol/L.

Usual Dose: See Package Insert.

LyphoMed, Inc., Rosemont, IL 60018   **B-87**

d.

5 mL DOSETTE® AMPUL   A-1416c

DOPAMINE
HCl INJECTION, USP

200 mg/5 mL

(40 mg/mL equivalent to 32.3 mg base)

FOR IV INFUSION ONLY
POTENT DRUG: MUST DILUTE BEFORE USING

esi ELKINS-SINN, INC.
CHERRY HILL, NJ 08003

LOT

e.

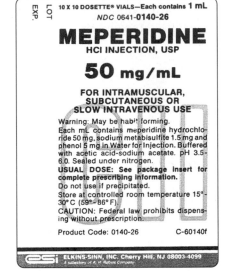

f.

N 0071–4200–03

Pitressin®
(Vasopressin
Inj, USP)
Synthetic
20 units
IM or SC use
1 mL
PARKE-DAVIS

4200G073

g.

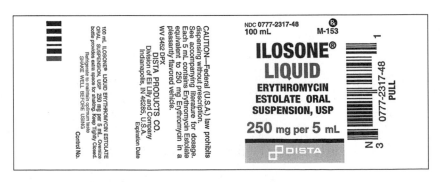

h.

FIGURE 13-33   Labels a and c courtesy of SmithKline Beecham Pharmaceuticals. Label g courtesy of Warner Lambert.

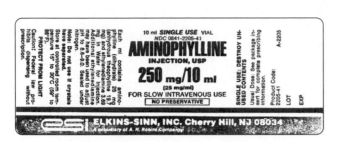

i.

j.

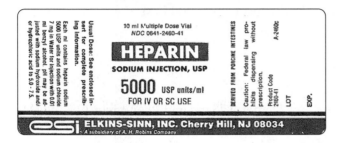

k.

l.

m.

FIGURE 13-33 *Continued*

195. Order: Chlorpromazine HCl 35 mg po

196. Order: Demerol (meperidine) 35 mg IM

197. Order: Aminophylline 150 mg IV

198. **Order:** Oxytetracycline 100 mg IM

199. **Order:** Dopamine HCl 125 mg IV

200. **Order:** H.P. Acthar Gel (corticotropin) 70 U IM

201. The patient is to receive Demerol 75 mg and Phenergan 12.5 mg IM in the same syringe.
    Label: Demerol (meperidine hydrochloride) 50 mg/mL
            Phenergan (promethazine hydrochloride) 25 mg/mL
    How many mL would contain the total amount of medication ordered?

202. A child weighing 35 lb is to receive Monistat i.v. (miconazole) 15 mg/kg IV q 8 hr. How many mg of Monistat will be administered in 24 hrs?

203. The patient is to receive Tagamet 800 mg per day to be divided in equal doses and given q 6 hr.
    Label: Tagamet (cimetidine hydrochloride) 300 mg/2 mL
    How many mL should be administered per dose?

204. The patient is to receive 125 mL/hr of 0.9% NS IV. How many mL/min will be administered?

205. The patient is to receive Lipo-Hepin 8000 units sc.
Label: Lipo-Hepin (heparin sodium) 10,000 U/mL
How many mL should be given?

206. An infant weighing 20 lb is to receive Gantricin 75 mg/kg/day in 4
divided doses po.
Label: Gantricin (sulfisoxazole) 0.5 g/tsp
How many mL should be given per dose?

207. The patient is to receive 1000 mL 5% D/W IV. How many g of glucose does the solution contain?

208. The patient has an IV of 1000 mL D5W to which Potassium Chloride 10 mEq is to be added.
Label: Potassium Chloride 2 mEq/mL
How many mL of KCl should be added to the IV solution?

209. The patient is to receive Pitocin (oxytocin) 5 units in 500 mL
Ringer's lactate solution IV. How many milliunits (mU) of Pitocin
does one mL of the solution contain?

210. The patient is to receive NegGram Suspension 2 g per day po in
equal doses q 6 hr.
Label: NegGram (naladaxic acid) 250 mg/tsp
How many mL should each dose contain?

211. The patient is to receive 500 mL of 25% D/W. How many kcal of Dextrose would the patient be receiving?

212. A patient weighing 160 lb is to receive Dobutrex (dobutamine hydrochloride) 7.5 mcg (μg)/kg/min IV. How many μg/hr will the patient receive?

213. The patient is to receive 750 mL of 5% D/NS in 5 hours. How many mL/hr should the patient receive?

214. The patient receives a total daily dosage of 2 g Chloromycetin po in equal doses q 6 hr.
Label: Chloromycetin (chloramphenicol) 250 mg/cap
How many capsules should the patient receive per dose?

215. The patient is to receive Revimine (dopamine hydrochloride) 400 mg in 1000 mL D5W IV to be administered at a rate of 5 mcg/kg/min.
How many mcg of Revimine does 1 mL of solution contain?

216. A patient weighing 150 lb is to receive Dopastat (dopamine hydrochloride) 400 mg in 500 mL of IV solution to be administered at a rate of 5 mcg/kg/min. How many mL/hr should the patient receive?

217. The patient is to receive Ritodrine Hydrochloride 150 mg in 500 mL of 5% Dextrose solution to infuse at a rate of 0.2 mg/min. How many mL/hr should be administered to infuse the ordered dose?

218. A child weighing 75 lb is to receive Morphine Sulfate 0.1 mg/kg of body weight sc.
Label: Morphine Sulfate 5 mg/mL
How many mL should be administered?

219. The patient is to receive Kefzol (cefazolin sodium) 8 g IM in 24 hrs to be given in equal doses at 6 hr intervals. How many mg should be administered per dose?

220. The patient is receiving an IV to which a piggyback of 100 mL of medication is to be added. The IVPB is to be infused in 45 min.
Drop Factor: 60 microdrops/mL
How many microdrops will be administered/min?

(**Note:** See Appendix G for answer key.)

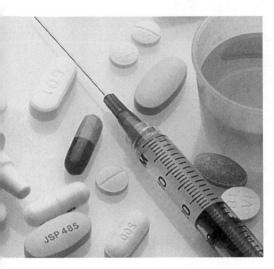

Arithmetic Review

Roman Numerals

RULE

1. Letters are used to designate numbers.
   I = 1
   V = 5
   X = 10
   L = 50
   C = 100
2. Reading from left to right:
   (a) if the first Roman numeral is greater than the following numeral(s), then add (all together).

EXAMPLE   VI = 5 + 1 = 6
               XII = 10 + 2 = 12

   (b) if the first Roman numeral is less than the following numeral(s), then subtract (smaller from the larger).

EXAMPLE   IV = 5 – 1 = 4
               XL = 50 – 10 = 40

   (c) if a smaller Roman numeral comes between 2 larger ones, subtract, then add.

EXAMPLE   XIV = 10 + (5–1) = 10 + 4 = 14
               LIX = 50 + (10–1) = 50 + 9 = 59

A. Express the following Arabic numerals as Roman numerals.

1. 6	**6.** 46
2. 50	**7.** 17
3. 3	**8.** 38
4. 12	**9.** 25
5. 24	**10.** 9

B. Express the following Roman numerals as Arabic numerals.

1. XLVII	**6.** VII
2. XXIX	**7.** II
3. V	**8.** LXVI
4. CXII	**9.** CCCIX
5. MCMXXXIII	**10.** XIII

Addition

Add the following whole numbers.

1.
$$\begin{array}{r} 12 \\ +16 \\ \hline \end{array}$$

2.
$$\begin{array}{r} 22 \\ +3 \\ \hline \end{array}$$

3.
$$\begin{array}{r} 43 \\ +15 \\ \hline \end{array}$$

4.
$$\begin{array}{r} 28 \\ 48 \\ +69 \\ \hline \end{array}$$

5.
$$\begin{array}{r} 39 \\ 88 \\ +16 \\ \hline \end{array}$$

6.
$$\begin{array}{r} 642 \\ 91 \\ +357 \\ \hline \end{array}$$

7.
$$\begin{array}{r} 611 \\ 292 \\ +386 \\ \hline \end{array}$$

8.
$$\begin{array}{r} 81 \\ 648 \\ +43 \\ \hline \end{array}$$

9.
$$\begin{array}{r} 8397 \\ 184 \\ +5240 \\ \hline \end{array}$$

10.
$$\begin{array}{r} 31,017 \\ 13 \\ +2,377 \\ \hline \end{array}$$

11. 6 + 23 =

12. 13 + 52 =

13. 19 + 32 + 15 =

14. 17 + 231 + 92 =

15. 700 + 26 + 845 =

16. 9 + 47 + 299 =

17. 393 + 209 + 567 =

18. 2,091 + 581 + 6,727 =

19. 8 + 5,496 + 745 =

20. 40 + 50,008 + 9,833 =

Subtraction

Subtract the following whole numbers.

1.
$$\begin{array}{r} 29 \\ -6 \\ \hline \end{array}$$

2.
$$\begin{array}{r} 215 \\ -38 \\ \hline \end{array}$$

3.
$$\begin{array}{r} 5309 \\ -342 \\ \hline \end{array}$$

4.
$$\begin{array}{r} 7333 \\ -4281 \\ \hline \end{array}$$

5.
$$\begin{array}{r} 73 \\ -41 \\ \hline \end{array}$$

6.
$$\begin{array}{r} 303 \\ -55 \\ \hline \end{array}$$

7.
$$\begin{array}{r} 12,965 \\ -492 \\ \hline \end{array}$$

8.
$$\begin{array}{r} 138 \\ -25 \\ \hline \end{array}$$

9.
$$\begin{array}{r} 8846 \\ -8721 \\ \hline \end{array}$$

10. $\begin{array}{r} 965 \\ -\ 82 \\ \hline \end{array}$

11. 42 − 31 =

12. 54 − 36 =

13. 235 − 66 =

14. 465 − 203 =

15. 209 − 65 =

16. 6699 − 301 =

17. 1124 − 908 =

18. 1865 − 1392 =

19. 32,945 − 2,030 =

20. 56,841 − 32,931 =

Multiplication   Multiply the following numbers.

1. $\begin{array}{r} 8 \\ \times 4 \\ \hline \end{array}$

2. $\begin{array}{r} 24 \\ \times 13 \\ \hline \end{array}$

3. $\begin{array}{r} 311 \\ \times 252 \\ \hline \end{array}$

4. $\begin{array}{r} 15 \\ \times 9 \\ \hline \end{array}$

5. $\begin{array}{r} 143 \\ \times 91 \\ \hline \end{array}$

6. $\begin{array}{r} 609 \\ \times 23 \\ \hline \end{array}$

7. $\begin{array}{r} 497 \\ \times 704 \\ \hline \end{array}$

8. $\begin{array}{r} 2536 \\ \times\ 219 \\ \hline \end{array}$

9. $\begin{array}{r} 1551 \\ \times\ 69 \\ \hline \end{array}$

10. $\begin{array}{r} 733 \\ \times 300 \\ \hline \end{array}$

11. 19 × 4 =

12. 21 × 6 =

13. 34 × 12 =

14. 62 × 18 =

15. 256 × 79 =

16. 689 × 203 =

17. 181 × 117 =

18. 1598 × 200 =

19. 18,452 × 1,501 =

20. 986 × 1000 =

Division   Solve the following division problems. Carry answers to two decimal places and round to nearest tenth.

1. $4\overline{)20}$

2. $25\overline{)295}$

3. $8\overline{)164}$

4. $3\overline{)925}$

5. $13\overline{)2363}$

6. $16\overline{)5493}$

7. $232\overline{)2696}$

8. $473\overline{)9652}$

9. $281\overline{)6795}$

10. $596\overline{)9235}$

11. 105 ÷ 5 =

12. 648 ÷ 8 =

13. 2222 ÷ 11 =

14. 6950 ÷ 30 =

15. 6393 ÷ 16 =

16. 15,321 ÷ 35 =

17. 16,209 ÷ 10 =

18. 18,492 ÷ 933 =

19. 802,495 ÷ 436 =

20. 111,666 ÷ 606 =

Fractions   **A.** Reduce the following fractions to lowest terms.

RULE

> Divide both numerator and denominator by the largest whole number that will go evenly into each.

EXAMPLE $\dfrac{5}{10} = \dfrac{5 \div 5}{10 \div 5} = \dfrac{1}{2}$

PRACTICE

1. $\dfrac{2}{6}$

2. $\dfrac{3}{9}$

3. $\dfrac{4}{8}$

4. $\dfrac{3}{15}$

5. $\dfrac{5}{55}$

6. $\dfrac{12}{48}$

7. $\dfrac{9}{10}$

8. $\dfrac{14}{56}$

9. $\dfrac{18}{80}$

10. $\dfrac{255}{1530}$

B. Convert the following mixed numbers to improper fractions.

RULE

> Multiply the whole number by the denominator, add to numerator, and place this sum over the original denominator.

EXAMPLE $5\dfrac{3}{8} = 5 \times 8 = 40 + 3 = \dfrac{43}{8}$

PRACTICE

1. 2 ¾   6. 9 ⅖

2. 7 ⁸⁄₉   7. 1 ⅔

3. 5 ³⁄₁₀   8. 1 ½

4. 12 ¼   9. 10 ⅖

5. 6 ⅔   10. 8 ³⁄₆

C. Convert the following improper fractions to mixed numbers. Reduce the fraction to lowest terms.

RULE

Divide the denominator into the enumerator and reduce to lowest terms.

EXAMPLE $\dfrac{72}{9} = 72 \div 9 = 8$

$\dfrac{45}{6} = 45 \div 6 = 7\dfrac{3}{6} = 7\dfrac{1}{2}$

PRACTICE

1. $\dfrac{25}{6}$ 3. $\dfrac{94}{5}$

2. $\dfrac{19}{3}$ 4. $\dfrac{62}{8}$

5. $\dfrac{16}{11}$

6. $\dfrac{40}{13}$

7. $\dfrac{122}{9}$

8. $\dfrac{125}{23}$

9. $\dfrac{82}{4}$

10. $\dfrac{99}{2}$

D. Add the following fractions. Convert answer to mixed numbers when possible and reduce fraction to lowest terms.

RULE

> When the denominators are the same, add the numerators and place this sum over the original denominator.

EXAMPLE

$$\begin{aligned} &\frac{1}{8} \\ +&\frac{3}{8} \\ \hline &\frac{4}{8} = \frac{1}{2} \end{aligned}$$

RULE

> 1. When the denominators are not the same, determine the least common denominator (LCD) by finding the smallest number divisible by both denominators.
> 2. Divide each denominator by this LCD and multiply each numerator by its respective quotient.
> 3. Add the numerators, place over the LCD and reduce to lowest terms.

EXAMPLE

$$\begin{aligned} \frac{2}{16} &= \frac{2}{16} \\ +\frac{1}{8} &= +\frac{2}{16} \qquad \text{LCD} = 16 \\ \hline &\quad \frac{4}{16} = \frac{1}{4} \end{aligned}$$

$$\begin{array}{rcl} \dfrac{7}{10} & = & \dfrac{49}{70} \\[2ex] +\dfrac{9}{35} & = & +\dfrac{18}{70} \quad \text{LCD} = 70 \\[2ex] & & \dfrac{67}{70} \end{array}$$

PRACTICE

1. $\dfrac{7}{9}$
    $+\dfrac{4}{9}$

2. $\dfrac{3}{4}$
    $+\dfrac{1}{4}$

3. $\dfrac{2}{6}$
    $+\dfrac{5}{6}$

4. $\dfrac{1}{12}$
    $+\dfrac{4}{12}$

5. $\dfrac{1}{15}$
    $\dfrac{2}{15}$
    $+\dfrac{6}{15}$

6. $\dfrac{32}{90}$
    $+\dfrac{16}{90}$

7. $\dfrac{1}{3}$
    $+\dfrac{3}{4}$

8. $\dfrac{2}{5}$
    $\dfrac{6}{10}$
    $+\dfrac{3}{5}$

9. $\dfrac{2}{3}$
    $\dfrac{5}{6}$
    $+\dfrac{4}{6}$

10. $\dfrac{60}{48}$
    $+\dfrac{34}{48}$

11. $\dfrac{1}{2} + \dfrac{2}{2} =$

12. $\dfrac{2}{3} + \dfrac{1}{3} =$

13. $\dfrac{5}{8} + \dfrac{2}{8} =$

14. $\dfrac{2}{3} + \dfrac{1}{4} + \dfrac{5}{6} =$

15. $\dfrac{2}{12} + \dfrac{3}{18} + \dfrac{2}{2} =$

16. $\dfrac{2}{3} + \dfrac{5}{12} + \dfrac{2}{4} =$

17. $\dfrac{3}{15} + \dfrac{10}{60} + \dfrac{1}{12} =$

18. $\dfrac{1}{4} + \dfrac{16}{64} + \dfrac{8}{32} =$

19. $\dfrac{9}{10} + \dfrac{20}{100} + \dfrac{6}{10} =$

20. $\dfrac{32}{18} + \dfrac{1}{18} + \dfrac{9}{72} =$

E. Subtract the following fractions. Convert answer to mixed numbers when possible and reduce fraction to lowest terms.

RULE

> When the denominators are the same, subtract the numerators and place this difference over the original denominator.

EXAMPLE

$$\begin{array}{r} \dfrac{7}{10} \\ -\dfrac{3}{10} \\ \hline \dfrac{4}{10} = \dfrac{2}{5} \end{array}$$

RULE

> 1. When the denominators are not the same, determine the least common denominator (LCD) by finding the smallest number divisible by both denominators.
> 2. Divide each denominator by this LCD and multiply each numerator by its respective quotient.
> 3. Subtract the numerators, place over the LCD and reduce to lowest terms.

EXAMPLE

$$\begin{array}{r} \dfrac{13}{21} \\ -\dfrac{4}{21} \\ \hline \dfrac{9}{21} = \dfrac{3}{7} \end{array}$$

PRACTICE

1. $\dfrac{5}{6}$
    $-\dfrac{1}{6}$

2. $\dfrac{3}{7}$
    $-\dfrac{2}{7}$

3. $\dfrac{7}{14}$
    $-\dfrac{3}{14}$

4. $\dfrac{3}{4}$
    $-\dfrac{2}{4}$

5. $\dfrac{19}{36}$
    $-\dfrac{6}{36}$

6. $\dfrac{9}{11}$
    $-\dfrac{2}{33}$

7. $\dfrac{10}{2}$
    $-\dfrac{4}{5}$

8. $\dfrac{90}{10}$
    $-\dfrac{12}{6}$

9. $\dfrac{36}{7}$
    $-\dfrac{2}{3}$

10. $\dfrac{50}{10}$
    $-\dfrac{30}{40}$

11. $\dfrac{2}{4} - \dfrac{1}{4} =$

12. $\dfrac{8}{12} - \dfrac{3}{12} =$

13. $\dfrac{4}{8} - \dfrac{3}{8} =$

14. $\dfrac{5}{8} - \dfrac{1}{2} =$

15. $\dfrac{14}{18} - \dfrac{6}{24} =$

16. $\dfrac{32}{8} - \dfrac{2}{4} =$

17. $\dfrac{100}{50} - \dfrac{3}{5} =$

18. $\dfrac{20}{15} - \dfrac{4}{5} =$

19. $\dfrac{28}{7} - \dfrac{2}{3} =$

20. $\dfrac{14}{2} - \dfrac{4}{6} =$

F. Multiply the following fractions. Convert answer to mixed numbers when possible and reduce fraction to lowest terms.

RULE

> 1. Convert mixed numbers to improper fractions.
> 2. Use cancellation and division to reduce the size of numbers in numerators or denominators.
> 3. Multiply numerators and denominators and reduce resulting fraction to lowest terms or convert to mixed number.

EXAMPLES

$$\frac{1}{\cancel{6}_{2}} \times \frac{\cancel{3}^{1}}{5} = \frac{1}{10} \qquad 2\frac{3}{4} \times 4\frac{1}{2} = \frac{11}{4} \times \frac{9}{2} = \frac{99}{8} = 12\frac{3}{8}$$

Hints on cancellation:

1. Look for powers of 10 (cross out zero(s))

EXAMPLES

a. $175,\cancel{000} \times \dfrac{1}{200,\cancel{000}} \quad$ (Divide by 5) $\quad = \dfrac{7}{8}$

(with $\cancel{35}^{7}$ above and $\cancel{40}\;8$ below) (then by another 5)

OR

$\cancel{175,000}^{7} \times \dfrac{1}{\cancel{200,000}\;8} \quad$ (Divide by 25) $\quad = \dfrac{7}{8}$

OR

b. $\cancel{290} \times \dfrac{1}{\cancel{1000}\;1} \times \dfrac{\cancel{500}}{\cancel{50}\;1} \times \dfrac{\cancel{60}^{10}}{1}^{1} = 29 \times 6 = 174$

Cross out zeros

OR

$\cancel{290}^{58} \times \dfrac{1}{\cancel{1000}\;2} \times \dfrac{\cancel{500}^{1}}{\cancel{50}\;1} \times \dfrac{\cancel{60}}{1} = 58 \times 6 = \dfrac{348}{2} = 174$

2. Any even numbers—such as 58, 2, or 6—can always be divided by 2.

EXAMPLE

$$\overset{58}{\cancel{290}} \times \frac{1}{\underset{\underset{1}{2}}{\cancel{1000}}} \times \frac{\overset{1}{\cancel{500}}}{\cancel{50}} \times \frac{\overset{3}{\cancel{60}}}{1} = 58 \times 3 = 174 \quad \textbf{OR} \quad 29 \times 6 = 174$$

either divide the 2 into 6 or 2 into 58

3. If the sum of the digits in a number can be divided by a certain number, then that number divides into the original number.

EXAMPLE

$$84 \times \frac{1}{2.2} \times \frac{8}{1} \times \frac{\overset{1}{\cancel{5}}}{\underset{15}{\cancel{75}}} \times \frac{5}{1}$$

If the sum of the digits in a number can be divided by 3, then 3 divides into the original number.

84 is 8 + 4 = 12

since 12 ÷ 3 is 4 (not a fraction)

then
$$\begin{array}{r} 28 \\ 3\overline{)84} \\ \underline{6} \\ 24 \\ \underline{24} \end{array}$$

$$\overset{28}{\cancel{84}} \times \frac{1}{2.2} \times \frac{8}{1} \times \frac{\overset{1}{\cancel{5}}}{\underset{\underset{1}{\underset{\cancel{5}}{\cancel{15}}}}{\cancel{75}}} \times \frac{\overset{1}{\cancel{5}}}{1}$$

now divide 28 or 8 and 2.2 by 2 (Example shows 8 and 2.2 divided by 2)

$$\overset{28}{\cancel{84}} \times \frac{1}{\underset{1.1}{\cancel{2.2}}} \times \frac{\overset{4}{\cancel{8}}}{1} \times \frac{\overset{1}{\cancel{5}}}{\underset{\underset{\cancel{5}}{\underset{1}{\cancel{15}}}}{\cancel{75}}} \times \frac{\overset{1}{\cancel{5}}}{1} = \frac{112}{1.1} = 1.1\overline{)112.0.000}$$

$$\begin{array}{r} 101.818 \\ 1.1\overline{)112.0.000} \\ \underline{11} \\ 20 \\ \underline{11} \\ 90 \\ \underline{88} \\ 20 \\ \underline{11} \\ 90 \end{array}$$

$$\frac{112}{1.1} = 102$$

or 101.8

or 101.82

1. $\dfrac{6}{7} \times \dfrac{3}{5} =$

2. $\dfrac{1}{4} \times \dfrac{3}{5} =$

3. $\dfrac{8}{10} \times \dfrac{1}{4} =$

4. $6\dfrac{2}{3} \times 5\dfrac{1}{2} =$

5. $5 \times 3\dfrac{2}{10} =$

6. $9 \times 3\dfrac{2}{3} =$

7. $6\dfrac{3}{7} \times 8 =$

8. $3\dfrac{2}{5} \times 20 =$

9. $4\dfrac{1}{6} \times 5\dfrac{1}{4} =$

10. $2\dfrac{6}{10} \times 1\dfrac{9}{10} =$

G. Divide the following fractions. Convert answer to mixed numbers when possible and reduce fraction to lowest terms.

RULE

1. Convert mixed numbers to improper fractions.
2. Invert the second fraction.
3. Cancel numerator and denominator wherever possible.
4. Multiply numerator and denominator and reduce resulting fraction to lowest terms or convert to mixed number.

EXAMPLE

$$\dfrac{1}{10} \div \dfrac{35}{5} = \dfrac{1}{\overset{}{\underset{2}{10}}} \times \dfrac{\overset{1}{\cancel{5}}}{3} = \dfrac{1}{6}$$

$$5\dfrac{3}{4} \div 3\dfrac{1}{6} = \dfrac{23}{\underset{2}{\cancel{4}}} \times \dfrac{\overset{3}{\cancel{6}}}{19} = \dfrac{69}{38} = 1\dfrac{31}{38}$$

1. $\dfrac{1}{4} \div \dfrac{2}{16} =$

2. $\dfrac{1}{2} \div \dfrac{3}{2} =$

3. $\dfrac{3}{6} \div \dfrac{22}{23} =$

4. $\dfrac{32}{4} \div 2 =$

5. $6\dfrac{2}{4} \div 4 =$

6. $2\dfrac{2}{5} \div 1\dfrac{3}{15} =$

7. $4\dfrac{2}{4} \div 3\dfrac{1}{2} =$

8. $2\dfrac{2}{8} \div 3\dfrac{4}{8} =$

9. $4\dfrac{6}{18} \div \dfrac{4}{8} =$

10. $20\dfrac{1}{2} \div 6\dfrac{1}{6} =$

> **Note:** When multiplying complex fractions, it is necessary to use both the multiplication and division rules for fractions.

EXAMPLES   **a.** $\dfrac{1}{6} \times \dfrac{20}{1/4} \times \dfrac{1}{15}$

Take $\dfrac{20}{1/4}$ to the side and get a simpler fraction.

$\dfrac{20}{1/4}$ means 20 divided by 1/4 or

$20 \div \dfrac{1}{4} = 20 \times \dfrac{4}{1} = 80$

So, $\dfrac{1}{6} \times \dfrac{20}{1/4} \times \dfrac{1}{15}$ becomes $\dfrac{1}{\underset{3}{6}} \times \overset{\overset{8}{16}}{80} \times \dfrac{1}{\underset{3}{15}} = \dfrac{8}{9}$

or 0.889 or 0.89 or 0.9

OR change $\dfrac{1}{4}$ to 0.25

$\dfrac{1}{6} \times \dfrac{20}{1/4} \times \dfrac{1}{15} = \dfrac{1}{\underset{3}{6}} \times \dfrac{\overset{\overset{2}{4}}{20}}{.25} \times \dfrac{1}{\underset{3}{15}} = \dfrac{2}{2.25}$

$$2.25\overline{)2.00.00}^{.88}$$
$$\underline{180}$$
$$2000$$
$$\underline{1800}$$

b. $\dfrac{1}{100} \times \dfrac{1}{1/150} \times \dfrac{15}{1}$

$1 \div \dfrac{1}{150} = 1 \times \dfrac{150}{1} = 150$

$= \dfrac{1}{\underset{2}{\cancel{100}}} \times \dfrac{\overset{3}{\cancel{150}}}{1} \times \dfrac{15}{1} = \dfrac{45}{2} = 22.5$

OR change $\dfrac{1}{150}$ to a decimal as shown in previous example

$\dfrac{1}{100} \times \dfrac{1}{1/150} \times \dfrac{15}{1}$

$\dfrac{1}{150} = 150\overline{)\underset{\displaystyle \begin{array}{l} \underline{900} \\ 1000 \\ \underline{900} \end{array}}{\overset{.0066}{1.0000}}}$

Because $\dfrac{1}{150}$ equals a repeating decimal, it is not a good idea to use this method here.

Note: To multiply fractions containing decimals in numerator or denominator, see the following examples.

EXAMPLES   **a.** $0.2 \times \dfrac{1000}{1} \times \dfrac{1}{400}$

Divide 200 into 1000 and 400

$0.2 \times \dfrac{\overset{5}{\cancel{1000}}}{1} \times \dfrac{1}{\underset{2}{\cancel{400}}}$

either divide 2 into 0.2 (see section on dividing decimals)

$2\overline{)\overset{.1}{.2}}$

$\overset{0.1}{\cancel{0.2}} \times \dfrac{\overset{5}{\cancel{1000}}}{1} \times \dfrac{1}{\underset{\underset{1}{\cancel{2}}}{\cancel{400}}} = 0.5$

OR

multiply 0.2×5 to 1.0 (see section on multiplying decimals)

$$0.2 \times \frac{\overset{5}{\cancel{1000}}}{1} \times \frac{1}{\underset{2}{\cancel{400}}}$$

$$1.0 \times \frac{1}{2} = \frac{1}{2}$$

b. $.006 \times \dfrac{\overset{15}{\cancel{60}}}{1} \times \dfrac{1}{\underset{.1}{\cancel{0.4}}}$ divide 4 into 60 and 0.4

$$= \frac{.090}{0.1} = 0.9 \qquad \begin{array}{r} 15 \\ \times .006 \\ \hline .090 \end{array} \qquad \begin{array}{r} .90 \\ .1\overline{)0.90} \\ 9 \\ \hline \end{array} \quad \text{or } 0.9$$

c. $\overset{3}{\cancel{150}} \times \dfrac{1}{\underset{2}{\cancel{1000}}} \times \dfrac{1}{\underset{0.25}{\cancel{0.75}}} \times \dfrac{\overset{1}{\cancel{30}}}{1} = \dfrac{3}{.50} = 6 \quad \begin{array}{r} 6 \\ .50\overline{)3.00} \\ 300 \\ \hline \end{array}$

Decimals   **A.** Write the following decimals in numbers.

RULE

Whole numbers are placed to the left of the decimal point; decimal fractions* are placed to the right of the decimal point.
*A decimal fraction is defined by its location to the right of the decimal point (e.g., one place = tenths, two places = hundredths, three places = thousandths, four places = ten-thousandths).

EXAMPLE   one and two tenths = 1.2
three and five hundredths = 3.05

Note: The decimal point is read as "and."

PRACTICE

1. twenty-four and two tenths

2. ten and four tenths

3. sixteen and twenty-nine hundredths

4. thirty and fifteen hundredths

5. two hundred sixty-one thousandths

6. three and three thousandths

7. nine ten-thousandths

8. thirty-two and twenty-seven ten-thousandths

9. six hundred-thousandths

10. twenty-five and eighty-five hundred-thousandths

B. Change the following decimals to fractions.

RULE

1. The numerator consists of the number(s) to the right of the decimal point.
2. The denominator consists of the decimal fraction (i.e., number of places to the right of the decimal point).

   EXAMPLE   1 = tenths (10), 2 = hundredths (100), etc.

   Note: The number of zeros in the denominator is always the same as the number of digits in the numerator.

EXAMPLE $0.1 = \dfrac{1}{10}$ $0.01 = \dfrac{1}{100}$

PRACTICE

1. 0.5   **3.** 0.53

2. 0.4   **4.** 0.25

5. 0.16   **8.** 0.973

6. 0.35   **9.** 0.4535

7. 0.548   **10.** 0.7246

C. Change the following fractions to decimals. Carry each answer to two decimal places and round to the nearest tenth.

RULE

Divide the numerator by the denominator.

EXAMPLE $\dfrac{5}{8} = 5 \div 8 = $ $8\overline{)5.000}$ ... .625

$$\begin{array}{r} .625 \\ 8\overline{)5.000} \\ \underline{48} \\ 20 \\ \underline{16} \\ 40 \\ \underline{40} \end{array}$$

$\dfrac{5}{8} = 0.625$ or 0.6 to nearest tenth

or 0.63 to nearest hundredth

PRACTICE

1. $\dfrac{1}{3}$ **6.** $\dfrac{12}{14}$

2. $\dfrac{1}{6}$ **7.** $\dfrac{8}{16}$

3. $\dfrac{2}{5}$ **8.** $\dfrac{5}{12}$

4. $\dfrac{5}{6}$ **9.** $\dfrac{1}{4}$

5. $\dfrac{3}{4}$ **10.** $\dfrac{14}{35}$

D. Add the following decimals.

RULE

> 1. Place decimals to be added in a column with decimal points one under the other.
> 2. Add the columns and place the decimal point directly under the line of decimal points.

EXAMPLE

$$
\begin{array}{r}
0.4 \\
+8.95 \\
\hline
9.35
\end{array}
$$

PRACTICE

1.
$$
\begin{array}{r}
0.2 \\
+1.76 \\
\hline
\end{array}
$$

2.
$$
\begin{array}{r}
.50 \\
22.80 \\
+\ 7.00 \\
\hline
\end{array}
$$

3.
$$
\begin{array}{r}
.30 \\
3.615 \\
+11.2 \\
\hline
\end{array}
$$

4.
$$
\begin{array}{r}
16. \\
2.345 \\
0.750 \\
+12.000 \\
\hline
\end{array}
$$

5.
$$
\begin{array}{r}
13.2 \\
6.215 \\
7.20 \\
+185.6 \\
\hline
\end{array}
$$

6.
$$
\begin{array}{r}
9.276 \\
10.31 \\
146.200 \\
+\ \ 8.3 \\
\hline
\end{array}
$$

7.
$$
\begin{array}{r}
6.03 \\
28.1 \\
7.2106 \\
+\ 48.1 \\
\hline
\end{array}
$$

8.
$$
\begin{array}{r}
2470.50316 \\
4.3922 \\
61.74 \\
+\ \ \ \ .111 \\
\hline
\end{array}
$$

9.
$$
\begin{array}{r}
0.000396 \\
21.25976 \\
8.71 \\
+\ \ 6.31256 \\
\hline
\end{array}
$$

10.
$$
\begin{array}{r}
62.132 \\
7.9204 \\
9.1 \\
168.0074 \\
+\ \ \ \ .2183 \\
\hline
\end{array}
$$

E. Subtract the following decimals.

RULE

> 1. Place the decimals to be subtracted in a column with decimal points one under the other.
> 2. Subtract the columns and place the decimal point directly under the line of decimal points.

EXAMPLE

$$
\begin{array}{r}
0.300^* \\
-\,0.106 \\
\hline
0.194
\end{array}
$$

*Zeros may be added after the decimal point without changing the value.

PRACTICE

1. $\begin{array}{r} 28.25 \\ -\ 6.10 \\ \hline \end{array}$

2. $\begin{array}{r} 386.152 \\ -\ 4.06 \\ \hline \end{array}$

3. $\begin{array}{r} 5.6 \\ -\ 3.92 \\ \hline \end{array}$

4. $\begin{array}{r} 92.0064 \\ -\ 2.84 \\ \hline \end{array}$

5. $\begin{array}{r} 201.6002 \\ -\ 29.364 \\ \hline \end{array}$

6. $\begin{array}{r} 0.921 \\ -\ 0.070352 \\ \hline \end{array}$

7. $\begin{array}{r} 24.92 \\ -\ 8.0286 \\ \hline \end{array}$

8. $\begin{array}{r} 17 \\ -\ 6.2813 \\ \hline \end{array}$

9. $\begin{array}{r} 793 \\ -\ 24.008 \\ \hline \end{array}$

10. $\begin{array}{r} 693.4228 \\ -\ 16.111 \\ \hline \end{array}$

F. Round off the following decimals to the place indicated.

RULE

> 1. Carry computation to one decimal place beyond the desired place.
> 2. If the final digit is 4 or less, leave prior digit the same.
> 3. If the final digit is 5 or more, increase the prior digit by 1.

EXAMPLE   Round to the nearest tenth:
$$7.01 = 7$$
Round to the nearest hundredth.
$$10.106 = 10.11$$

PRACTICE

1. 2.32 to nearest tenth

2. 3.44 to nearest tenth

3. 32.66 to nearest tenth

4. 16.791 to nearest hundredth

5. 41.105 to nearest hundredth

6. 15.4038 to nearest hundredth

7. 3.2896 to nearest thousandth

8. 291.6345 to nearest thousandth

9. 782.5211 to nearest tenth

10. 2.6859 to nearest tenth

G. Multiply the following decimals.

RULE

> **1.** Multiply as whole numbers.
> **2.** Count the total number of decimal places in the problem.
> **3.** Starting from the right, count off the same number of places in the answer.
> **4.** If necessary, add zeros to provide enough places in the answer.

EXAMPLE

$$
\begin{array}{r}
3.9 \quad \text{(1 decimal place)} \\
\times\ 0.005 \quad \text{(3 decimal places)} \\
\hline
0.0195 \quad \text{(4 decimal places)}
\end{array}
$$

PRACTICE

1. $\begin{array}{r} 16.3 \\ \times\ 0.8 \\ \hline \end{array}$

2. $\begin{array}{r} 32.6 \\ \times 0.25 \\ \hline \end{array}$

3. $\begin{array}{r} 93.6 \\ \times\ 3.2 \\ \hline \end{array}$

4. $\begin{array}{r} 17.81 \\ \times\ 6.02 \\ \hline \end{array}$

5. $\begin{array}{r} 71.3 \\ \times 84.2 \\ \hline \end{array}$

6. $\begin{array}{r} 0.025 \\ \times\ 0.2 \\ \hline \end{array}$

7. $\begin{array}{r} 0.087 \\ \times\ 0.6 \\ \hline \end{array}$

8. $\begin{array}{r} 0.09302 \\ \times\ \ \ \ 2.4 \\ \hline \end{array}$

9. $\begin{array}{r} 0.234 \\ \times\ \ \ \ 7 \\ \hline \end{array}$

10. $\begin{array}{r} 2.361 \\ \times\ \ \ \ 9 \\ \hline \end{array}$

H. Divide the following decimals. Carry to two decimal places and round to the nearest tenth.

RULE

> 1. If the divisor is a whole number, proceed as in division of whole numbers. In the answer, place the decimal point directly above its position in the dividend.
> 2. If the divisor is a decimal, move the decimal point to the right end, making the divisor a whole number. Move the decimal point in the dividend the same number of places to the right (adding zeros if necessary). Then proceed as in division of whole numbers.

EXAMPLE

$$
\begin{array}{r}
3\ 33.33 \\
0.24\overline{)80.00.00} \\
\underline{72} \\
80 \\
\underline{72} \\
80 \\
\underline{72} \\
80 \\
\underline{72} \\
80 \\
\underline{72} \\
8
\end{array}
$$

PRACTICE

1. $2.5\overline{)100.0}$

2. $3.24\overline{)9.1006}$

3. $0.6\overline{)1.75}$

4. $2.0\overline{)9.0}$

5. $7.3\overline{)62.59}$

6. $0.423 \div 3 =$

7. $1.5 \div 0.5 =$

8. $326.5 \div 22 =$

9. $222 \div 0.11 =$

10. $1.843 \div 20 =$

(**Note:** See Appendix G for answer key.)

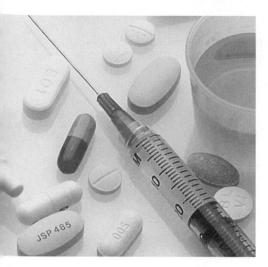

APPENDIX B

Conversion between Celsius and Fahrenheit Temperatures

Although electronic digital thermometers are replacing the use of glass thermometers in health-care settings, the latter are still commonly enough used that health-care workers should be able to convert between Celsius and Fahrenheit temperatures. Figure B-1 compares these two scales.

Note that the Fahrenheit degree is smaller than the Celsius, i.e., 180 Fahrenheit degrees between the boiling and freezing points of water, as compared to 100 degrees on the Celsius. The factor 1.8 is used to convert from one degree size to the other.

It can be seen that 0°C is not the same as 0°F. In fact, 32°F = 0°C. The factor 32 is used to account for the different zero points.

FIGURE B-1   Fahrenheit Celsius scales

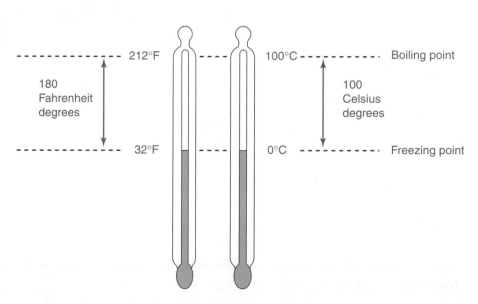

From this information, the following formulas have been derived for converting between the two scales.

$$C° = \frac{F° - 32}{1.8}$$
$$F° = 1.8\ C° + 32$$

Obviously, either formula can be used to determine either C or F, so only one need be memorized.

EXAMPLE Convert 101°F to C

$$C = \frac{F - 32}{1.8}$$
$$C = \frac{101 - 32}{1.8}$$
$$C = 38.3°$$

EXAMPLE Convert 42°C to F
$$F = 1.8\ C + 32$$
$$F = 1.8 \times 42 + 32$$
$$F = 107.6°$$

PRACTICE
Convert the following temperatures, rounding answers to tenths.

1. 104°F = _____ C

2. 28°C = _____ F

3. 99°F = _____ C

4. 9°C = _____ F

5. 110°F = _____ C

6. 37°C = _____ F

7. 95°F = _____ C

8. 52°C = _____ F

9. 98.6°F = _____ C

10. 34°C = _____ F

(**Note:** See Appendix G for answer key.)

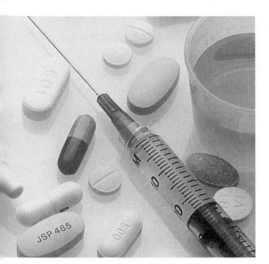

APPENDIX C

Measuring and Recording Fluid Balance

Accurate measurement and recording of fluid intake and output is an important aspect of health care. Intake consists of all fluids ingested by mouth or by tube feeding plus fluids given parenterally, i.e., IV. Output consists of urine excreted plus fluids lost during emesis and diarrhea, if measurable. In addition, diaphoresis and rapid breathing should be noted in the medical record as these are forms of fluid loss that are not typically measured but should be documented.

Measurements are recorded in cc (mL) or oz, depending on hospital policy, on some type of fluid balance sheet.

A. Calculate the total fluid intake in mL for 24 hours and record below.

Breakfast	6 ounces milk
	4 ounces apple juice
	4 ounces water
	450 mL 5% D/W IV
Lunch	6 ounces soup
	6 ounces coffee
	4 ounces ice cream
Snack	6 ounces ginger ale
	5 ounces water
Dinner	6 ounces vegetable juice
	6 ounces milk
	5 ounces coffee
	4 ounces gelatin

Snack 4 ounces sherbet

     8 ounces water

     500 mL 5% D/W IV

Night 6 ounces water

     550 mL Lactated Ringers IV

          Total = _____ mL

B. Calculate the total fluid output in mL for 24 hours and record below.

  7–3 400 cc

     300 cc

     250 cc

  3–11 200 cc

     300 cc

     250 cc

  11–7 250 cc

     350 cc

     300 cc

          Total = _____ mL

(**Note:** See Appendix G for answer key.)

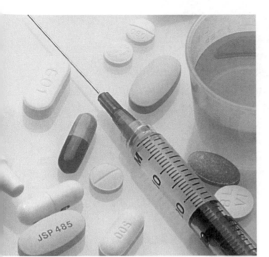

Dimensional Analysis Variation

Some students who have previously learned the technique of dimensional analysis have been taught to identify as starting factor the desired unit to which the known quantity will be converted, preceded by a question mark.

EXAMPLE   Express 1.32 yards in inches.

First, write down the desired unit preceded by a question mark. Then, set it equal to the known quantity.

$$? \text{ inches} = 1.32 \text{ yards}$$

Then, choose appropriate units for conversion factors that will lead from the given units (yards) to the desired units (inches).

$$\text{yards} \rightarrow \text{feet} \rightarrow \text{inches}$$
$$(\text{or yards} \rightarrow \text{inches})$$

$$? \text{ inches} = 1.32 \text{ yards} \times \frac{3 \text{ feet}}{1 \text{ yard}} \times \frac{12 \text{ inches}}{1 \text{ foot}} = 47.52 \text{ inches}$$

$$(\text{or } ? \text{ inches} = 1.32 \text{ yards} \times \frac{36 \text{ inches}}{1 \text{ yard}} = 47.52 \text{ inches})$$

It can be seen that since ? inches and 1.32 yards are equivalent values, interchanging them as starting factor and answer unit does not change the result; therefore the practice is acceptable.

Furthermore, some students may have been taught that it is not necessary to arrange corresponding units sequentially (diagonally) in the conversion equation so that cancellable labels are in sequential conversion factors. The rationale for this is that as long as conversion factors remain 1:1 relationships, the placement of factors does not affect the result. The writers feel that this practice increases the chance for error and should be discouraged. It is strongly recommended that conversion factors be arranged as taught in Step II of dimensional analysis methodology in Chapter I, so that units are cancelled sequentially in a consistent manner until the desired unit for the answer, which is in the final conversion factor, is reached.

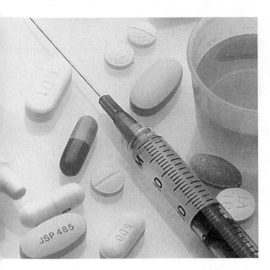

Twenty-Four Hour Clock

Most health-care institutions are using the 24-hour clock for documenting medication administration, especially with the use of computerized MARs. The chance for error is greatly reduced because the same numbers are never repeated.

EXAMPLE

	AM	PM
Traditional time	10	10
24-hour time	1000	2200

Refer to Figure E-1

FIGURE E-1   24-hour clock

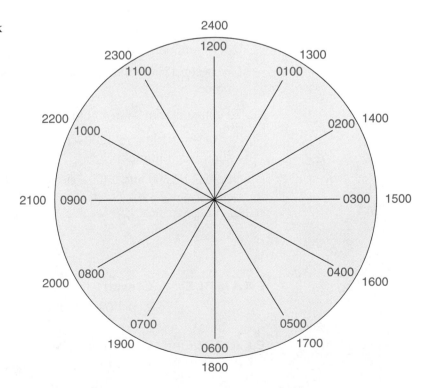

The inside numbers represent the hours from 1:00 A.M. to 12 noon (A.M. time). The outside numbers represent the hours between 1:00 P.M. and midnight (P.M. time).

From 12 midnight to 1:00 A.M., the time is stated in minutes, e.g., 0001, 0002, 0015, 0030, etc., to 0059. After 0059, hours are stated in 100s, e.g., 0100 (1 A.M.), 0200 (2 A.M.), etc., to 2400 (midnight). See Table E-1.

TABLE E-1   Comparison of Traditional and 24-Hour Clocks

A.M.		P.M.	
Traditional	24-Hour	Traditional	24-Hour
12 midnight	02400	12 noon	1200
1	0100	1	1300
2	0200	2	1400
3	0300	3	1500
4	0400	4	1600
5	0500	5	1700
6	0600	6	1800
7	0700	7	1900
8	0800	8	2000
9	0900	9	2100
10	1000	10	2200
11	1100	11	2300

RULE

To convert from traditional to 24-hour clock:

between 1:00 A.M. and 12 noon—delete the colon and precede single digit numbers with a zero.

between 12 noon and 12 midnight—add 12 hours to the traditional time.

To convert from 24-hour clock to traditional:

between 0100 and 1200—replace colon and drop zero preceding single digit numbers.

between 1300 and 2400—subtract 1200 (12 hours) and replace the colon.

EXAMPLE   Convert 9:00 A.M. to 24-hour time

9:00 = 0900 hours

EXAMPLE   Convert 1:15 P.M. to 24-hour time

1:15 + 1200 = 1315 hours

EXAMPLE   Convert 0100 hours to traditional time
0100 = 1:00 A.M.

EXAMPLE   Convert 2030 hours to traditional time
2030 − 1200 = 8:30 P.M.

PRACTICE
Convert traditional to 24-hour time

1. 3:00 P.M. = _____

2. 10:00 A.M. = _____

3. 5:00 P.M. = _____

4. 12 midnight = _____

5. 9:30 P.M. = _____

6. 7:00 A.M. = _____

7. 9:00 P.M. = _____

8. 10:00 P.M. = _____

9. 8:00 A.M. = _____

10. 6:15 P.M. = _____

Convert 24-hour time to traditional time

1. 0016 hours = _____

2. 0815 hours = _____

3. 1700 hours = _____

4. 2015 hours = _____

5. 2245 hours = _____

6. 1030 hours = _____

7. 0800 hours = _____

8. 1115 hours = _____

9. 1200 hours = _____

10. 0930 hours = _____

(**Note:** See Appendix G for answer key.)

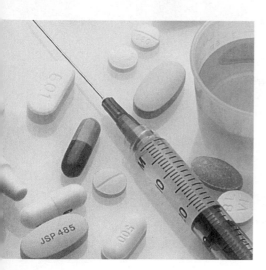

APPENDIX F

Percentage Solutions

A solution is a liquid preparation containing one or more dissolved or diluted substances. The diluting fluid is called the *solvent* and the drug or other substance being dissolved is called the *solute.*

To prepare a specified percentage strength of a solution, it is necessary to calculate the exact amount of drug that must be added to a certain volume of liquid to produce a solution of the desired strength.

As a rule, percentage solutions are prepared by the pharmacist if they are not commercially available. Occasionally, it may be necessary for the nurse to prepare a percentage solution to be used for patient care or for disinfection (e.g., mouth rinse, throat irrigation, wet dressing, enema, douche) or for terminal disinfection of hospital equipment and contaminated areas. Dimensional analysis can be used to calculate the amounts of solvent and solute necessary to prepare these solutions.

Equivalent Units for Solids and Liquids

In solutions, the word percent or the symbol % means the *parts of substance per 100 parts of solution.* For example, 2% indicates two parts of 100 parts total. The measured parts either must be units of the *same kind* or else must be *equivalents.* Certainly 2 grams of salt in 100 pounds of mixture could not be called a 2% mixture as grams and pounds are not equivalent units. The parts can be minims, drams, fluid ounces, cups, milliliters, or liters, for instance. For example, a 10% solution of alcohol means 10 parts of alcohol to 100 parts of solution. Because they are both liquids, the parts that measure both the alcohol and the total solution would be of the same kind. For instance, the solution could have 10 minims of alcohol for 100 minims of solution, 10 fluid ounces of alcohol for 100 fluid ounces of solution, or 10 pints of alcohol for 100 pints of solution. However, if a dry substance were to be placed into solution, equivalent units relating dry measure to liquid measure must be used. For example, a 5% salt solution would require 5 grains of salt for 100 minims of solution, 5 grams of salt for 100 milliliters of solution, or 5 ounces of salt for 100 fluid ounces of solution. It is important in this case to know the equivalents for dry and liquid measure, which are listed below.

Equivalents

Dry Units	Fluid Units
grain	minim
gram	milliliter
dram	fluid dram
ounce	fluid ounce
kilogram	liter

Calculation of Percentage Solutions Using Dimensional Analysis

The percentage strength of a desired solution is expressed as a conversion factor that contains the relationship between solute and solvent.

EXAMPLE Find the quantity of alcohol needed to prepare 200 mL of a 15% alcohol solution. The parts (solute and solvent) will be measured in mL. The conversion factor can be written as:

$$\frac{15 \text{ mL alcohol}}{100 \text{ mL solution}} \quad \text{or} \quad \frac{100 \text{ mL solution}}{15 \text{ mL alcohol}}$$

Problem: Find the quantity of alcohol needed to prepare 200 mL of solution.

Definite quantity: 200 mL of solution. This is the starting factor and the problem proceeds as follows:

Starting Factor	Answer Unit
200 mL solution	mL alcohol

Equivalent: 15 mL alcohol = 100 mL solution

Conversion Equation:

$$200 \text{ mL solution} \times \frac{15 \text{ mL alcohol}}{100 \text{ mL solution}} = 30 \text{ mL alcohol}$$

(**Note:** In this problem, not only are the units labeled as mL but also the substances are clearly identified.)

REMEMBER
It is extremely important that the quantity of total solution is not confused with the quantity of substance dissolved; therefore, the descriptive label should be used.

EXAMPLE Find the quantity of 25% solution needed to supply 15 grains of drug.

Starting Factor	Answer Unit
gr 15 drug	ɱ solution

Equivalent: 25 gr drug = 100 ɱ solution

Conversion Equation:

$$15 \; \cancel{\text{gr drug}} \times \frac{100 \; \text{ɱ solution}}{25 \; \cancel{\text{gr drug}}} = 60 \; \text{ɱ solution}$$

(**Note:** In the second factor, grains of drug has to appear in the denominator to *cancel the label* of the first factor. However, the relationship 100 minims of solution to 25 grains of drug is an equivalent expression and gives a true relationship even when inverted.)

EXAMPLE   Find the number of grams of dry drug needed to prepare 60 mL of 5% solution.

Starting Factor	Answer Unit
60 mL solution	g drug

Equivalent: 5 g drug = 100 mL solution

Conversion Equation:

$$60 \; \cancel{\text{mL solution}} \times \frac{5 \; \text{g drug}}{100 \; \cancel{\text{mL solution}}} = 3 \; \text{g}$$

EXAMPLE   Find the volume of 10% solution that can be made using four 5-grain tablets of drug.

Starting Factor	Answer Unit
4 tablets	ɱ solution

Equivalents: 5 gr drug = 1 tab, 10 gr drug = 100 ɱ solution

Conversion Equation:

$$4 \; \cancel{\text{tabs}} \times \frac{5 \; \cancel{\text{gr drug}}}{1 \; \cancel{\text{tab}}} \times \frac{100 \; \text{ɱ solution}}{10 \; \cancel{\text{gr drug}}} = 200 \; \text{ɱ solution}$$

EXAMPLE   Find the number of 10 grain tablets needed to make a pint of 2% solution of drug.

Starting Factor	Answer Unit
1 pt solution	tablets

Equivalents: 1 pt = 1 oz, 2 oz drug = 100 oz solution, 1 oz = 8 ʒ, 1 ʒ = 60 gr, 10 gr = 1 tab

Conversion Equation:

$$1 \; \cancel{\text{pt solution}} \times \frac{16 \; \cancel{\text{oz}}}{1 \; \cancel{\text{pt}}} \times \frac{2 \; \cancel{\text{oz drug}}}{100 \; \cancel{\text{oz solution}}} \times \frac{8 \; \cancel{\text{dr}}}{1 \; \cancel{\text{oz}}} \times \frac{60 \; \cancel{\text{gr}}}{1 \; \cancel{\text{dr}}} \times \frac{1 \; \text{tab}}{10 \; \cancel{\text{gr}}} = 15.3$$

or 15 tablets

EXAMPLE   Prepare 2500 mL of a 1:1000 solution using 1 g tablets.

Starting Factor	Answer Unit
2500 mL solution	tablets

Equivalents: 1 g = 1000 mL, 1 g = 1 tab

Conversion Equation:

$$2500 \; \cancel{\text{mL solution}} \times \frac{1 \; \cancel{\text{g drug}}}{1000 \; \cancel{\text{mL solution}}} \times \frac{1 \; \text{tab}}{1 \; \cancel{\text{g drug}}} = 2.5 \; \text{tablets}$$

(**Note:** Solution strength may be expressed either as percentage or as a ratio. The ratio 1:1000 means there is one part solute in 1000 parts of solvent and the conversion factor in the above problem is written as

$$\frac{1 \; \text{g drug}}{1000 \; \text{mL solution}} \; . \;)$$

Self-Quiz—Equivalents   Match dry units with equivalent fluid units.

_____ 1. grain   **A.** fluid dram

_____ 2. gram   **B.** fluid ounce

_____ 3. dram   **C.** liter

_____ 4. ounce   **D.** milliliter

_____ 5. kilogram   **E.** minim

PRACTICE
Calculation of Percentage Solutions

1. How many mL of solute are needed to prepare 4000 mL of a 2% Lysol solution?

2. How many grams of solute are needed to prepare 2 oz of 8% iodine solution?

3. Prepare 1000 mL of 70% alcohol solution.

4. Prepare 1000 mL of 1% Neomycin solution from 5 g Neomycin tablets.

5. Prepare 4000 mL 1:1000 bichloride of mercury solution using 500 mg tablets.

6. Prepare 500 mL 1:2000 potassium permanganate solution using potassium permanganate crystals (measure in g).

7. Prepare 1000 mL 1:100 potassium permanganate solution using potassium permanganate crystals (measure in g).

8. Prepare 250 mL 1% acetic acid solution from a 10% solution.

9. Prepare 2000 mL of 1:1000 bichloride of mercury solution using 0.5 g tablets.

10. How many mL of alcohol are needed to prepare 1 qt of 40% alcohol solution?

Answer Key   **Self-Quiz—Equivalents (page 319)**

1. E
2. D
3. A
4. B
5. C

Practice: Calculation of Percentage Solutions (pages 319–320)

1. 80 mL Lysol/3920 mL water
2. 4.8 g iodine
3. 700 mL alcohol/300 mL water
4. 2 Neomycin tab/1000 mL water
5. 8 bichloride of mercury tab/4000 mL water
6. 0.25 g potassium permanganate crystals/500 mL water
7. 10 g potassium permanganate crystals/1000 mL water
8. 25 mL acetic acid/225 mL water
9. 4 bichloride of mercury tab/2000 mL water
10. 400 mL alcohol/600 mL water

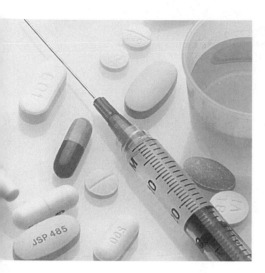

APPENDIX G

Answer Keys

**Chapter 1
Dimensional Analysis**

Practice: Identifying the Starting Factor and Answer Unit (page 4–5)

	STARTING FACTOR	ANSWER UNIT
1.	3 gr 3	mg
2.	5 kg	lb
3.	250 mg	tab
4.	0.5 g	cap
5.	250 mg	mL
6.	650 pennies	quarters
7.	9 dimes	nickels
8.	5.08 cm	inches
9.	26.2 mi	kilometers
10.	350 mi	dollars

Practice: Identifying Equivalents (page 8)

1. 3 ft = 1 yd
2. 12 in = 1 ft
3. 4 quarters = 1 dollar
4. 2 nickels = 1 dime
5. 2.5 cm = 1 in
6. 60 mg = 1 gr 1
7. 2.2 lb = 1 kg
8. 1000 mg = 1 g
9. 1000 mg = 1 g
10. 5 mL = 1 tsp

Practice: Setting Up Conversion Equations
(pages 12–13)

1. Equivalents: 500 mg = 1 tsp, 1 tsp = 5 mL

   Conversion Equation: $250 \text{ mg} \times \dfrac{1 \text{ tsp}}{500 \text{ mg}} \times \dfrac{5 \text{ mL}}{1 \text{ tsp}} = $ _____ mL

2. Equivalents: 250 mg = 5 mL

   Conversion Equation: $125 \text{ mg} \times \dfrac{5 \text{ mL}}{250 \text{ mg}} = $ _____ mL

3. Equivalents: 0.5 g = ʒ 1, ʒ 1 = 4 mL

   Conversion Equation: $0.75 \text{ g} \times \dfrac{ʒ 1}{0.5 \text{ g}} \times \dfrac{4 \text{ mL}}{ʒ 1} = $ _____ mL

4. Equivalents: gr 1 = 60 mg, 1 tab = 15 mg

   Conversion Equation: gr $\tfrac{1}{8} \times \dfrac{60 \text{ mg}}{\text{gr } 1} \times \dfrac{1 \text{ tab}}{15 \text{ mg}} = $ _____ tab

5. Equivalents: 5 mL = 1 tsp, 1 tsp = 300 mg

   Conversion Equation: $15 \text{ mL} \times \dfrac{1 \text{ tsp}}{5 \text{ mL}} \times \dfrac{300 \text{ mg}}{1 \text{ tsp}} = $ _____ mg

6. Equivalents: 12 in = 1 ft

   Conversion Equation: $84 \text{ in} \times \dfrac{1 \text{ ft}}{12 \text{ in}} = $ _____ ft

7. Equivalents: 2.2 lb = 1 kg

   Conversion Equation: $6.5 \text{ lb} \times \dfrac{1 \text{ kg}}{2.2 \text{ lb}} = $ _____ kg

8. Equivalents: 1 oz = 30 mL

   Conversion Equation: $675 \text{ mL} \times \dfrac{1 \text{ oz}}{30 \text{ mL}} = $ _____ oz

9. Equivalents: 1 L = 1000 mL

   Conversion Equation: $2.5 \text{ L} \times \dfrac{1000 \text{ mL}}{1 \text{ L}} = $ _____ mL

10. Equivalents: 5 mL = 1 tsp

    Conversion Equation: $10 \text{ mL} \times \dfrac{1 \text{ tsp}}{5 \text{ mL}} = $ _____ tsp

**Practice: Solving Conversion Equations
(pages 15–17)**

1. Equivalents: 0.125 mg = 1 tab

   Conversion Equation: $0.250 \, \text{mg} \times \dfrac{1 \, \text{tab}}{0.125 \, \text{mg}} = 2 \, \text{tab}$

2. Equivalents: 30 mg = 1 cap, 60 mg = gr 1

   Conversion Equation: $\text{gr} \, \frac{1}{2} \times \dfrac{60 \, \text{mg}}{\text{gr} \, 1} \times \dfrac{1 \, \text{cap}}{30 \, \text{mg}} = 1 \, \text{cap}$

3. Equivalents: 0.5 g = 1 tab, 1000 mg = 1 g

   Conversion Equation: $250 \, \text{mg} \times \dfrac{1 \, \text{g}}{1000 \, \text{mg}} \times \dfrac{1 \, \text{tab}}{0.5 \, \text{g}} = 0.5 \, \text{tab}$

4. Equivalents: gr ¼ = 1.4 mL

   Conversion Equation: $\text{gr} \, \frac{1}{6} \times \dfrac{1.4 \, \text{mL}}{\text{gr} \, \frac{1}{4}} = 0.9 \, \text{mL}$

5. Equivalents: gr ¹⁄₁₅₀ = 1 mL

   Conversion Equation: $\text{gr} \, \frac{1}{100} \times \dfrac{1 \, \text{mL}}{\text{gr} \, \frac{1}{150}} = 1.5 \, \text{mL}$

   OR

   $\text{gr} \, 0.01 \times \dfrac{1 \, \text{mL}}{\text{gr} \, 0.007} = 1.4 \, \text{mL}$

6. Equivalents: gr 7.5 = 5 mL, gr 15 = 1 g

   Conversion Equation: $1 \, \text{g} \times \dfrac{\text{gr} \, 15}{1 \, \text{g}} \times \dfrac{5 \, \text{mL}}{\text{gr} \, 7.5} = 10 \, \text{mL}$

7. Equivalents: 400 mg = 1 tsp, 5 mL = 1 tsp

   Conversion Equation: $10 \, \text{mL} \times \dfrac{1 \, \text{tsp}}{5 \, \text{mL}} \times \dfrac{400 \, \text{mg}}{1 \, \text{tsp}} = 800 \, \text{mg}$

8. Equivalents: 125 mg = 5 mL

   Conversion Equation: $200 \, \text{mg} \times \dfrac{5 \, \text{mL}}{125 \, \text{mg}} = 8 \, \text{mL}$

9. Equivalents: 30 mg = 5 mL

   Conversion Equation: $75 \, \text{mg} \times \dfrac{5 \, \text{mL}}{30 \, \text{mg}} = 12.5 \, \text{mL}$

10. Equivalents: gr 1 ½ = 1 tab, gr 1 = 60 mg

Conversion Equation: $90 \, \text{mg} \times \dfrac{\text{gr } 1}{60 \, \text{mg}} \times \dfrac{1 \text{ tab}}{\text{gr } 1.5} = 1 \text{ tab}$

Chapter 2
The Metric System of Measurement

Practice: Convert within the Metric System (page 23)

1. 3.2 L
2. 0.4 g
3. 2 kg
4. 5 mg
5. 0.3 m

6. 750 mL
7. 220 mg
8. 2500 g
9. 2.5 cm
10. 12,000 mcg

Chapter 3
The Apothecaries System of Measurement

Practice: Abbreviations (page 26)

1. ʒ
2. gr
3. ♍

4. s̄s̄
5. ℥

Practice: Convert Within the Apothecaries System (page 28)

1. 1 ⁷⁄₁₀ qt
2. ½ oz or ℥ s̄s̄
3. 24 oz or ℥ 24
4. ½ dr or ʒ s̄s̄
5. ½ dr or ʒ s̄s̄

6. 10 dr or ʒ x
7. ³⁄₁₀ oz or ℥ ³⁄₁₀
8. 256 dr or ʒ 256
9. 56 oz or ℥ 56
10. 3 ⁹⁄₁₀ lb

Chapter 4
The Household System of Measurement

Practice: Abbreviations (page 30)

1. gtt
2. gal
3. pt

4. tbs
5. tsp

Practice: Convert Within the Household System (page 32)

1. 48 tsp
2. 256 oz
3. 16 cups
4. 5.7 ft
5. 2 oz

6. 18 tsp
7. 2.8 gal
8. 8 tbs
9. 8.3 oz
10. 12 tbs

Chapter 5
Conversion of Metric, Apothecaries, and Household Units

Self-Quiz—Equivalents

A. Fill in the Blanks (page 33)

1. 1 gr 1		**6.** 1 gtt	
2. 1 g		**7.** 1000 mL	
3. 1000 mg		**8.** 2.5 cm	
4. 1000 g		**9.** 39.4 in	
5. 2.2 lb		**10.** ½ oz	

B. Match Equivalent Amounts (page 34)

1. d		**4.** b	
2. c		**5.** a	
3. e			

Practice (pages 37–38)

1. 1250 mL		**16.** 22.5 mL	
2. 88 lb		**17.** 480 mL	
3. 2.5 cups		**18.** ʒ 7.5	
4. 10 mL		**19.** 8 g	
5. 30 mg		**20.** 71.4 kg	
6. 1.4 kg		**21.** 180 mg	
7. 1.3 mL		**22.** 45 ♏	
8. 8 tbs		**23.** 11.4 lb	
9. ʒ 19.2		**24.** 12 cm	
10. gr 30		**25.** 24 in	
11. 90 gtt		**26.** ʒ 64	
12. 75 ♏		**27.** gr 1.5	
13. gr 2		**28.** gr 82.5	
14. 0.7 mL		**29.** 4 tbs	
15. 2.5 tsp		**30.** 300 mg	

Chapter 6
Calculation of Oral Medications

Practice: Reading Labels (pages 44–46)

A. Figure 6-6

1. Inderal LA 80		**5.** Ayerst	
2. propranolol hydrochloride		**6.** 1	
3. 80 mg/cap		**7.** 2	
4. capsule			

B. Figure 6-7

1. None		**5.** Roxane	
2. Potassium Chloride		**6.** 11.25 mL	
3. 15 mEq/11.25 mL		**7.** 7.5 mL	
4. liquid			

C. Figure 6-8

    1. Nitrostat

    2. Nitroglycerin

    3. 0.6 mg (gr $\frac{1}{100}$)/tab

    4. Sublingual tablet

    5. Parke-Davis

D. Figure 6-9

    1. Restoril

    2. temazepam

    3. 15 mg/cap

    4. capsule

    5. Sandoz

Practice: Reading Labels and Clinical Calculations Involving Medications Administered by the Oral Route (po) (pages 47–49)

1. 2 tab

2. 2 tab

3. 12 mL

4. nystatin, 500,000 U

5. prochlorperazine maleate, 2 tab

Practice: Oral Dosage Based on Body Weight (page 51)

1. 2 tab

2. 3 cap

3. 14.6 mL

4. 4.5 tab

5. 2 tab

Practice: Clinical Calculations Involving Medications Administered by the Oral Route (po) (pages 52–64)

1. 2 cap	**17.** 0.5 tab	**33.** 1 tab
2. 2 tab	**18.** 2 dr	**34.** 1 cap
3. 2 tab	**19.** 15 mL	**35.** 2.5 mL
4. 4 tab	**20.** 14.1 mL	**36.** 1 cap
5. 4 cap	**21.** 3 tab	**37.** 8 mL
6. 2 tab	**22.** 3 tab	**38.** 4 tab
7. 2 cap	**23.** 2 cap	**39.** 0.5 tab
8. 1 cap	**24.** 6.8 mL	**40.** 1.5 tab
9. 6 mL	**25.** 10 mL	**41.** 2.5 mL
10. 2 cap	**26.** 3 tab	**42.** 2 tab
11. 3 tab	**27.** 0.5 tab	**43.** 4 mL
12. 6 mL	**28.** 0.25 tab	**44.** 3 tsp
13. 2 tab	**29.** 2 cap	**45.** 2.5 mL
14. 2.4 mL	**30.** 7.5 mL	**46.** 8 mL
15. 2 tab	**31.** 2 cap	**47.** 1.2 mL
16. 0.5 tab	**32.** 1 tab	**48.** 2 tab

49. 2 cap	**52.** 4 tab	**54.** 2 tab
50. 1 tab	**53.** 1 tab	**55.** 2 tab
51. 12.5 mL		

**Chapter 7
Administration of
Oral Medications**

Self-Quiz—Abbreviations (pages 69–70)

A. Match the abbreviations with correct meaning

1. c	**6.** l
2. b	**7.** f
3. i	**8.** n
4. e	**9.** h
5. a	**10.** d

B. Write the Term

1. before meals	**6.** without
2. capsule	**7.** elixir
3. gram	**8.** whenever necessary
4. after meals	**9.** one-half
5. every three hours	**10.** milliliter

C. Identify the Route

1. intramuscular	**6.** both eyes
2. intravenous	**7.** by mouth
3. subcutaneous	**8.** sublingual
4. left eye	**9.** intradermal
5. right eye	

Practice: Simulated Medication Administration using MAR (pages 80–82)

1.

Medication	Amount to be Given
Digoxin	0.25 mg
K-Lor	20 mEq
Alupent Syrup	1.5 tsp
Erythromycin D-R	500 mg
Haldol	1.5 mg or 0.75 mL

2. 2 tab at 7:30 A.M.

3. ■ water or juice
   ■ 120 mL

4. ■ 20 mg/tab
   ■ 1 tab

5. ■ 7.5 mL
   ■ 15 mg
   ■ yes

6. ■ 15 mL
   ■ 20 doses

7. ■ 100 mg/cap
   ■ 1 cap

8. ■ 4 mg
   ■ 2 mg

9. ■ Darvocet-N 100
   ■ every 4 hours as needed
   ■ 1 tab

**Chapter 8
Calculation of
Parenteral Medications**

Shade in the Dosage (page 88)

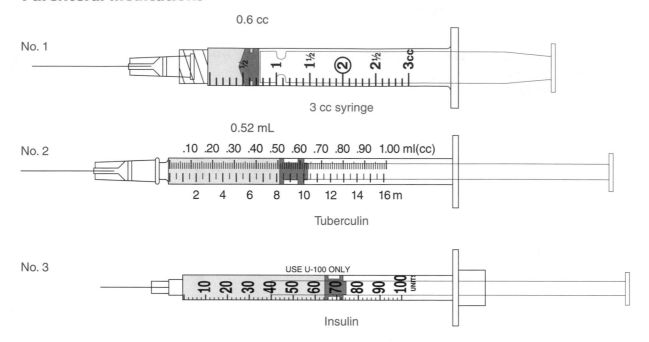

No. 1

0.6 cc

3 cc syringe

No. 2

0.52 mL

.10 .20 .30 .40 .50 .60 .70 .80 .90 1.00 ml(cc)

2 4 6 8 10 12 14 16 m

Tuberculin

No. 3

USE U-100 ONLY

10 20 30 40 50 60 70 80 90 100 UNITS

Insulin

Practice: Reading Labels (pages 94–97)

1. cyclophosphamide
   a. 1 g
   b. 50 mL
   c. 50 mL = 1 g
2. Moxam
   a. IV or IM
   b. 10 mL
   c. 270 mg = 1 mL
3. 20 mg
   a. 10 mg/mL
   b. gentamycin sulfate injection
   c. Schering
4. Cefazolin Sodium
   a. 2 mL
   b. 225 mg/mL
   c. refrigerator
5. IM
   a. 100 mg
   b. IM
   c. Vistaril

6. 2–12 g daily
   a. 5 mL
   b. 0.9% Sodium Chloride or 5% dextrose
   c. IV, IM, IP
7. Ceclor
   a. multiple
   b. 20 mg/kg/day in 3 divided doses
      250 mg tid
   c. 125 mg/5 mL
8. 10 mL
   a. 50 mg/cc
   b. oxytetracycline
   c. Roerig Pfizer
9. thiothixene Hcl
   a. IM
   b. no
   c. 2 mL

Practice: Calculating Dosages from Premixed Solutions (pages 99–105)

1. 0.6 mL
2. 1.5 mL, hydroxyzine hydrochloride
3. 1.5 mL or 1.7 mL
4. 0.5 mL, glycopyrrolate
5. 1.5 mL, penicillin G procaine
6. 0.6 mL, cefazolin sodium
7. 0.5 mL, kanamycin sulfate
8. 0.7 mL, dimenhydrinate
9. 0.5 mL, Lanoxin
10. 0.5 mL or 0.6 mL

11. 1.6 mL
12. 1.6 mL
13. 0.8 mL
14. 2 mL
15. 1 mL
16. 3 mL
17. 0.8 mL
18. 0.8 mL
19. 1.5 mL
20. 1 mL

Practice: IM Calculations Based on Body Weight (pages 106–107)

1. 1.9 mL
2. 3.3 mL
3. 1.2 mL
4. 2.2 mL
5. 2 mL

6. 1.4 mL
7. 2.5 mL
8. 0.8 mL
9. 1.2 mL
10. 1.5 mL

Practice: Medications Dispensed in Units (pages 109–111)

1. 0.4 mL
2. 0.7 mL
3. 1.7 mL
4. 0.8 mL
5. 0.8 mL

6. 0.75 mL
7. 1.7 mL
8. 1.1 mL
9. 0.1 mL
10. 0.3 mL

Practice: Reconstitution of Drugs in Powder Form (pages 114–120)

1. cefuroxime sodium
   a. 3.6 mL
   b. label
   c. 750 mg = 3.6 mL
   d. 2.4 mL
2. oxacillin
   a. sterile water for injection
   b. 5.7 mL

   c. 250 mg = 1.5 mL
   d. 1.8 mL
   e. 250–500 mg q 4–6 h
   f. ■ 10 A.M. on 9/19
      ■ 10 A.M. on 9/23
3. ticarcillin disodium
   a. sterile water for injection or 1% Lidocaine HCl sol (without epinephrine)

b. 1g/2.6 mL
c. 1.8 mL
d. IV
4. cephalothin sodium
   a. sterile water for injection
   b. 4 mL
   c. 0.5 g/2.2 mL
   d. 2.2 mL
   e. 2 g
   f. 2–12 g daily
   g. 9 A.M. on 11/13
   h. within 12 h
5. a. 2 mL
   b. 1.6 mL
   c. 0.8 mL
   d. 0.4 mL
   e. 1 week

f. refrigerator
6. 0.6 mL
7. 1.2 mL
8. 2.5 mL
9. 0.6 mL
10. 2 mL
11. 2.2 mL
12. 2 mL
13. 1 mL
14. 1.6 mL
15. 2 mL
16. 3 mL
17. 2.5 mL
18. 4.4 mL
19. 1.5 mL
20. 0.9 mL

Chapter 9
Administration of Parenteral Medications

Practice: Reading Insulin Labels (pages 139–142)

1. U 100
2. Lilly, Novo Nordisk
3. ■ a, b, f, g, j
  ■ f, g, i
  ■ l, m
  ■ d
  ■ e
  ■ e, k, l
4. ■ R
  ■ S
  ■ N
  ■ L

■ U
■ P
5. a. 1. a
    2. 24 units
  b. 1. h
    2. 45 units
  c. 1. d, m
    2. Regular
    3. 48 units
  d. 1. c, h
    2. Lente
    3. 66 units

Chapter 10
Calculation of Intravenous Medications and Solutions

Reading Labels: Drop Factor (page 152)

A. Figure 10-4
1. a. 10
  b. 15
  c. 60
2. a, b
3. c

Reading IV Labels (pages 152–153)

A. Figure 10-5
  1. 500 mL
  2. 5%
  3. Abbott
B. Figure 10-6
  1. 250 mL
  2. 0.9%

C. Figure 10-7
  1. 1000 mL
  2. 5%
  3. NaCl, NaLactate, KCl, CaCl

Practice: Calculation of IV Flow Rate When Total Infusion Time Is Specified (pages 161–162)

1. 31 gtt
2. 25 gtt
3. 50 gtt
4. 23 gtt
5. 35 gtt
6. 52 gtt
7. 28 gtt
8. 6 gtt
9. 100 gtt
10. 13 gtt

Practice: Calculation of IV Flow Rate When Infusion Rate Is Specified (pages 162–163)

11. 31 gtt
12. 17 gtt
13. 38 gtt
14. 21 gtt
15. 125 gtt
16. 20 gtt
17. 13 gtt

Practice: Calculation of Flow Rate When IV Contains Medication (pages 164–167)

1. 63 gtt
2. 125 gtt
3. 25 gtt
4. 50 gtt
5. 33 gtt

Practice: Calculation of the Number of mL/hr That Will Infuse (pages 166–167)

1. 125 mL
2. 83 mL
3. 125 mL
4. 125 mL
5. 104 mL
6. 83 mL
7. 125 mL

Practice: Calculation of Infusion Time (pages 168–169)

1. 12 hr 30 min
2. 8 hr 54 min
3. 4 hr
4. 14 hr 42 min
5. 7 hr 12 min

Practice: Adding Drugs to IVs and Calculating Flow Rate in gtt/min (pages 172–176)

1. cefazolin sodium
   a. 2 mL
   b. 1.6 mL
   c. 25 gtt
2. a. 2.4 mL
   b. 125 gtt
3. Omnipen-N
   a. 3 mL
   b. 38 gtt
4. a. 15 mL
   b. 28 gtt
5. a. 3 mL
   b. 150 gtt
6. 121 gtt
7. a. 1 mL
   b. 17 gtt
8. a. 1.3 mL
   b. 25 gtt
9. a. 3.1 mL
   b. 167 gtt
10. a. 10 mL
    b. 25 gtt

Practice: Calculation of the Volume of Solution or Concentration of Drug (pages 179–183)

1. a. 2.5 mL
   b. 100 mL
2. 25 mL
3. 8 mL
4. 50 mL
5. 100 mL
6. 100 mL
7. 121 mL
8. a. 6 mL
   b. 67 mL
9. a. 300 mL
   b. 10 min
10. 50 mg
11. 4 mg
12. 3 mcg
13. 1.25 mEq
14. 96 mg
15. a. 10 mL
    b. 267 mL
    c. 2 hr 54 min
16. a. 40 mL
    b. 0.13 g
    c. 400 mL
    d. 8 hr
17. a. 15 mL
    b. 0.3 mg
    c. 20 mL
    d. 30 mL
    e. 40 mL

**Practice: IV Flow Rate and Dosages Based on Body Weight
(pages 185–187)**

1. **a.** 459.1 mcg/min
   b. 55 mL/hr
   c. 55 gtt/min
   d. 8.3 mcg/gtt

2. **a.** 515.2 mcg/min
   b. 31 mL/hr
   c. 31 gtt/min
   d. 16.6 mcg/gtt

3. **a.** 135 mcg/min
   b. 41 mL/hr
   c. 41 gtt/min

   d. 3.3 mcg/gtt

4. **a.** 582.4 mcg/min
   b. 11 mL/hr
   c. 11 gtt/min
   d. 52.9 mcg/gtt

5. **a.** 416 mcg/min
   b. 15 mL/hr
   c. 15 gtt/min
   d. 27.7 mcg /gtt

Practice: Titration Infusions (pages 190–195)

1. **a.** 10,000 mcg/mL
   b. Lower: 3181.8 mcg/min
      Upper: 6363.6 mcg/min
   c. Lower: 19 mL/hr or 19
      gtt/min
      Upper: 38 mL/hr or 38
      gtt/min
   d. 167.5 mcg/gtt
   e. 4020 mcg/min

2. **a.** 800 mcg/mL
   b. Lower: 397.7 mcg/min
      Upper: 795.5 mcg/min
   c. Lower: 30 mL/hr or 30
      gtt/min
      Upper: 60 mL/hr or 60
      gtt/min
   d. 13.3 mcg/gtt
   e. 532 mcg/min

3. **a.** 5000 mcg/mL
   b. Lower: 350 mcg/min
      Upper: 700 mcg/min
   c. Lower: 4 mL/hr or 4
      gtt/min

      Upper: 8 mL/hr or 8
      gtt/min
   d. 87.5 mcg/gtt
   e. 787.5 mcg/min

4. **a.** 100 mcg/mL
   b. Lower: 136 mcg/min
      Upper: 272.7 mcg/min
   c. Lower: 82 mL/hr or 82
      gtt/min
      Upper: 164 mL/hr or 164
      gtt/min
   d. 1.7 mcg/gtt
   e. 130.9 mcg/min

5. **a.** 400 mcg/mL
   b. Lower: 150 mcg/min
      Upper: 375 mcg/min
   c. Lower: 23 mL/hr or 23
      gtt/min
      Upper: 56 mL/hr or 56
      gtt/min
   d. 6.5 mcg/gtt
   e. 182 mcg/min

Practice: IV Bolus (pages 196–200)

1. a. 0.8 mL
   b. 24 sec
2. a. 2 mL
   b. 2 min
3. a. 0.6 mL
   b. 1 min 12 sec
4. a. 3.5 mL
   b. 1 min 48 sec
5. a. 9.6 mL
   b. 9 min 36 sec

6. a. 306.8 mg
   b. 0.6 mL
   c. 12 min 18 sec
7. a. 77.3 mg
   b. 7.7 mL
   c. 2 min 12 sec
   d. 5 mL
   e. 30 mL

Practice: Nutrition Calculations (pages 202–203)

1. 255 kcal
2. 140 kcal
3. 110 kcal
4. 42.5 kcal
5. 420 kcal
6. 850 kcal

7. 600 kcal
8. 2040 kcal
9. a. 200 kcal
   b. 425 kcal
10. a. 170 kcal
    b. 340 kcal

Practice: Adjusting IVs (pages 205–208)

1. a. 35 gtt
   b. 33 gtt
2. a. 42 gtt
   b. 44 gtt
3. a. 42 gtt
   b. 33 gtt
4. a. 21 gtt
   b. 27 gtt
5. a. 63 gtt
   b. 50 gtt

6. a. 31 gtt
   b. 33 gtt
7. a. 28 gtt
   b. 32 gtt
8. a. 50 gtt
   b. 40 gtt
9. a. 35 gtt
   b. 31 gtt
10. a. 63 gtt
    b. 60 gtt

Chapter 12 Pediatric Dosage

Practice: Calculating Pediatric Dosage Based on Body Weight—Oral Medications (pages 221–224)

1. digoxin, 7.6 mL
2. 2.6 mL
3. 9.7 mL

4. 6.8 mL
5. 5.5 mL
6. 7.5 mL

7. 5 mL

8. 9.3 mL

9. 9.5 mL

10. 4.5 mL

11. 5.1 mL

12. 13.2 mL

13. 1.7 mL

14. 6.4 mL

15. 0.6 mL

Practice: Calculating Pediatric Dosage—Injections (pages 225–227)

1. Kantrex, 1 mL

2. furosemide, 3.4 mL

3. 0.75 mL

4. 0.27 mL

5. 2.5 mL

6. 0.12 mL

7. 0.59 mL

8. 1.1 mL

9. 2.3 mL

10. 0.045 mL or 0.05 mL

Practice: Calculating Pediatric Dosage—IVs (pages 229–232)

1. a. 7.5 mL

  b. 978 mcg

  c. 58.7 mg

  d. 49 mL

  e. 5 hr 6 min

2. a. 1.2 mL

  b. 37 mcg

  c. 2.2 mg

  d. 18 mL/hr or 19 mL/hr

3. a. 6.1 mg

  b. 0.24 mL

4. 0.36 mL

5. 3.3 mL

6. a. 12.1 mL

  b. 212 gtt

7. a. 0.76 mL

  b. 300 gtt

8. a. 0.87 mL

  b. 200 gtt

Practice: Use the Nomogram to Determine Child's BSA (pages 233–234)

1. $1.22 \, M^2$

2. $0.8 \, M^2$

3. $1.1 \, M^2$

4. $0.47 \, M^2$

5. $0.53 \, M^2$

Practice: Use Nomogram and Dimensional Analysis to Calculate Pediatric Dosages (pages 234–235)

1. 10.3 mg

2. 4.4 mg

3. 101.2 mg

4. 161.8 mg

5. 185.3 mg

Chapter 13
Clinical Calculations

Practice: Solve Using Dimensional Analysis (pages 237–283)

1. 2 cap
2. 0.5 tab
3. 0.5 tab
4. 10 mL
5. 2 cap
6. 2 tab
7. 2 cap
8. 3 tab
9. 12.5 mL
10. 2 tab
11. 2.5 mL
12. 6 mL
13. 2 cap
14. 2.5 mL
15. 2 tsp
16. 800 mg
17. 3 tab
18. 22.5 mL
19. ½ tab
20. 2 tab
21. 2.4 mL
22. 2 tab
23. 18 or 20 mL
24. 2 tab
25. 0.5 tab
26. 2 tab
27. 3 cap
28. 2 cap
29. 1 ½ tab
30. 3 tab
31. 4 tab
32. 2 tab
33. 1 tab
34. 10 mL
35. 2.5 mL
36. 10 mL
37. 1 tab
38. 2 cap
39. 0.5 tab

40. 4 tab
41. 2 tab
42. 3 cap
43. 12 mL
44. 2 tab
45. 4 tab
46. 1 tab
47. 1 tab
48. 10 mL
49. 1.3 mL
50. 1 mL
51. 1.7 mL
52. 0.5 mL
53. 0.8 mL
54. 1.4 mL
55. 1.2 mL
56. 0.75 mL
57. 0.6 mL
58. 1 mL
59. 1.5 mL
60. 4 ℳ
61. 0.5 mL
62. 0.5 mL
63. 0.4 mL
64. 1.8 mL
65. 4 mL
66. 0.6 mL
67. 0.67 mL
68. 0.76 mL
69. 0.72 mL
70. 0.6 mL
71. 1.6 mL
72. 0.5 mL
73. 0.5 mL
74. 0.7 mL
75. 4 mL
76. 0.8 mL
77. 0.6 mL
78. 0.56 mL

79. 1 or 1.1 mL
80. 0.67 mL
81. Give 1.3 mL, Discard 0.7 mL
82. 3 mL
83. 0.6 mL
84. 1.2 mL
85. 2.3 mL
86. 0.7 mL
87. 0.16 mL
88. 0.75 mL
89. 0.75 mL
90. 0.89 mL
91. 0.25 mL
92. 1.5 mL
93. 1.6 mL
94. 1.4 mL
95. 0.4 mL
96. 1.3 mL
97. 1.7 mL
98. 0.67 mL
99. 1.7 mL
100. 1 mL
101. 1.1 mL
102. 0.9 mL
103. 2.4 mL
104. 3 mL
105. 0.6 mL
106. 1.5 mL
107. 0.5 mL
108. 0.05 mL
109. 0.4 mL
110. 0.7 mL
111. 31 gtt
112. 31 gtt
113. 26 gtt
114. 42 gtt
115. 63 gtt
116. 31 gtt

117. 10 gtt

118. 36 gtt

119. 21 gtt

120. 6 gtt

121. 8 gtt

122. 28 gtt

123. 21 gtt

124. 38 gtt

125. 25 gtt

126. 36 gtt

127. 14 gtt

128. 42 gtt

129. 31 gtt

130. 83 gtt

131. 25 gtt

132. 42 gtt

133. 7 gtt

134. 150 gtt

135. **a.** 20 mL

    b. 100 gtt

136. **a.** 30 mL

    b. 10 gtt

137. 10 hr 24 min

138. **a.** 7 mL

    b. 100 gtt

139. 35 gtt

140. **a.** Add 21 mL

    b. 30 gtt

141. 100 gtt

142. **a.** 1.5 mL

    b. 10 gtt

143. **a.** Flow rate: 12 gtt

    b. 8 hr 18 min

144. 60 units

145. 30 gtt

146. **a.** 375 mcg/min

    b. 28 mL

    c. 28 gtt

    d. 13.4 mcg/gtt

147. **a.** 23.5 U/min

    b. 50 mL

    c. 50 gtt

148. **a.** 310.4 mcg/min

    b. 93 mL

    c. 93 gtt

    d. 3.3 mcg/gtt

149. **a.** 822.7 mcg/min

    b. 99 mL

    c. 99 gtt

    d. 8.3 mcg/gtt

150. **a.** 886 mcg/min

    b. 66 mL

    c. 66 gtt

    d. 13.4 mcg/gtt

151. **a.** 198.2 mcg/min

    b. 59 mL

    c. 59 gtt

    d. 3.4 mcg/gtt

152. **a.** 200 mcg/mL

    b. Lower: 45 mcg/min

    Upper: 135 mcg/min

    c. Lower: 14 mL/hr or 14 gtt/min

    Upper: 41 mL/hr or 41 gtt/min

    d. 3.2 mcg/gtt

    e. 60.8 mcg/min

153. 21 mL

154. **a.** 8 mL

    b. 25 gtt

155. 7 hr 6 min

156. **a.** 6 mL

    b. 106 gtt

157. **a.** 5.9 mL

    b. 100 gtt

158. **a.** 10 mL

    b. 28 gtt

159. 60 min

160. **a.** 150 gtt

    b. 75 gtt

161. 24,000 U

162. **a.** 1.5 mL

    b. 3 min

163. 70 mg

164. **a.** 7.5 mL

    b. 5 min

165. **a.** 1.1 mL

    b. 1 min 6 sec

166. **a.** 0.8 mL

    b. 0.32 min or 19 sec

167. 400 kcal

168. 170 kcal

169. 70 kcal

170. 165 kcal

171. 1 tab

172. 2.5 mL

173. 3 tab

174. 0.1 mL

175. 2 cap

176. 7 mL

177. 0.6 mL

178. 5 mL

179. 4.5 mL

180. 13.6 mL

181. 0.7 mL

182. **a.** 325 mcg/min

    b. 39 mL/hr

183. 6.2 mL

184. 0.68 mL

185. 7.7 mL

186. 32.9 mg

187. 1.9 mL

188. 0.16 mg

189. 0.07 mg

190. 0.38 mg

191. 0.65 mL	**201.** 2 mL	**211.** 500 kcal
192. 3 mL	**202.** 715.8 mg/24 hr	**212.** 32,730 μg
193. 0.4 mL	**203.** 1.3 mL/dose	**213.** 150 mL
194. 0.6 mL	**204.** 2 mL	**214.** 2 cap
195. 1.4 mL	**205.** 0.8 mL	**215.** 400 mcg
196. 0.7 mL	**206.** 1.7 mL	**216.** 26 mL
197. 6 mL	**207.** 50 g	**217.** 40 mL
198. 2 mL	**208.** 5 mL	**218.** 0.7 mL
199. 3.1 mL	**209.** 10 mU	**219.** 2000 mg
200. 0.88 mL	**210.** 10 mL	**220.** 133 gtt

Appendix A
Arithmetic Review

Roman Numerals (page 286)

A. Express as Roman Numerals

1. VI	**6.** XLVI
2. L	**7.** XVII
3. III	**8.** XXXVIII
4. XII	**9.** XXV
5. XXIV	**10.** IX

B. Express as Arabic Numerals

1. 47	**6.** 7
2. 29	**7.** 2
3. 5	**8.** 66
4. 112	**9.** 309
5. 1933	**10.** 13

Addition (page 286)

Add Whole Numbers

1. 28	**11.** 29
2. 25	**12.** 65
3. 58	**13.** 66
4. 145	**14.** 340
5. 143	**15.** 1571
6. 1090	**16.** 355
7. 1289	**17.** 1169
8. 772	**18.** 9399
9. 13,821	**19.** 6249
10. 33,407	**20.** 59,881

Subtraction (pages 286–287)

Subtract Whole Numbers

1. 23		**11.** 11	
2. 177		**12.** 18	
3. 4967		**13.** 169	
4. 3052		**14.** 262	
5. 32		**15.** 144	
6. 248		**16.** 6398	
7. 12,473		**17.** 216	
8. 113		**18.** 473	
9. 125		**19.** 30,915	
10. 883		**20.** 23,910	

Multiplication (page 287)

Multiply Numbers

1. 32		**11.** 76	
2. 312		**12.** 126	
3. 78,372		**13.** 408	
4. 135		**14.** 1116	
5. 13,013		**15.** 20,224	
6. 14,007		**16.** 139,867	
7. 349,888		**17.** 21,177	
8. 555,384		**18.** 319,600	
9. 107,019		**19.** 27,696,452	
10. 219,900		**20.** 986,000	

Division (page 287)

Division Problems

1. 5		**11.** 21	
2. 11.8		**12.** 81	
3. 20.5		**13.** 202	
4. 308.3		**14.** 231.7	
5. 181.8		**15.** 399.6	
6. 343.3		**16.** 437.7	
7. 11.6		**17.** 1620.9	
8. 20.4		**18.** 19.8	
9. 24.2		**19.** 1840.6	
10. 15.5		**20.** 184.3	

Fractions (pages 288–297)

A. Reduce to Lowest Terms

1. $\dfrac{1}{3}$ 6. $\dfrac{1}{4}$

2. $\dfrac{1}{3}$ 7. $\dfrac{9}{10}$

3. $\dfrac{1}{2}$ 8. $\dfrac{1}{4}$

4. $\dfrac{1}{5}$ 9. $\dfrac{9}{40}$

5. $\dfrac{1}{11}$ 10. $\dfrac{1}{6}$

B. Convert to Improper Fractions

1. $\dfrac{11}{4}$ 6. $\dfrac{47}{5}$

2. $\dfrac{71}{9}$ 7. $\dfrac{5}{3}$

3. $\dfrac{53}{10}$ 8. $\dfrac{3}{2}$

4. $\dfrac{49}{4}$ 9. $\dfrac{52}{5}$

5. $\dfrac{20}{3}$ 10. $\dfrac{51}{6}$

C. Convert to Mixed Numbers (reduce to lowest terms)

1. $4\dfrac{1}{6}$ 6. $3\dfrac{1}{13}$

2. $6\dfrac{1}{3}$ 7. $13\dfrac{5}{9}$

3. $18\dfrac{4}{5}$ 8. $5\dfrac{10}{23}$

4. $7\dfrac{3}{4}$ 9. $20\dfrac{1}{2}$

5. $1\dfrac{5}{11}$ 10. $49\dfrac{1}{2}$

D. Add Fractions (change to mixed numbers and reduce to lowest terms)

1. $\frac{11}{9} = 1\frac{2}{9}$

2. $\frac{4}{4} = 1$

3. $\frac{7}{6} = 1\frac{1}{6}$

4. $\frac{5}{12}$

5. $\frac{9}{15} = \frac{3}{5}$

6. $\frac{48}{90} = \frac{8}{15}$

7. $\frac{13}{12} = 1\frac{1}{12}$

8. $\frac{16}{10} = 1\frac{3}{5}$

9. $\frac{13}{6} = 2\frac{1}{6}$

10. $\frac{94}{48} = 1\frac{23}{24}$

11. $\frac{3}{2} = 1\frac{1}{2}$

12. $\frac{3}{3} = 1$

13. $\frac{7}{8}$

14. $\frac{21}{12} = 1\frac{3}{4}$

15. $\frac{48}{36} = 1\frac{1}{3}$

16. $\frac{19}{12} = 1\frac{7}{12}$

17. $\frac{27}{60} = \frac{9}{20}$

18. $\frac{48}{64} = \frac{3}{4}$

19. $\frac{170}{100} = 1\frac{7}{10}$

20. $\frac{141}{72} = 1\frac{23}{24}$

E. Subtract Fractions (change to mixed numbers and reduce to lowest terms)

1. $\frac{4}{6} = \frac{2}{3}$

2. $\frac{1}{7}$

3. $\frac{4}{14} = \frac{2}{7}$

4. $\frac{1}{4}$

5. $\frac{13}{36}$

6. $\frac{25}{33}$

7. $\frac{42}{10} = 4\frac{1}{5}$

8. $\frac{210}{30} = 7$

9. $\frac{94}{21} = 4\frac{10}{21}$

10. $\frac{170}{40} = 4\frac{1}{4}$

11. $\dfrac{1}{4}$

12. $\dfrac{5}{12}$

13. $\dfrac{1}{8}$

14. $\dfrac{1}{8}$

15. $\dfrac{114}{216} = \dfrac{19}{36}$

16. $\dfrac{28}{8} = 3\dfrac{1}{2}$

17. $\dfrac{70}{50} = 1\dfrac{2}{5}$

18. $\dfrac{8}{15}$

19. $\dfrac{70}{21} = 3\dfrac{1}{3}$

20. $\dfrac{38}{6} = 6\dfrac{1}{3}$

F. Multiply Fractions

1. $\dfrac{18}{35}$

2. $\dfrac{3}{20}$

3. $\dfrac{1}{5}$

4. $36\dfrac{2}{3}$

5. 16

6. 33

7. $51\dfrac{3}{7}$

8. 68

9. $21\dfrac{7}{8}$

10. $4\dfrac{47}{50}$

G. Divide Fractions

1. 2

2. $\dfrac{1}{3}$

3. $\dfrac{23}{44}$

4. 4

5. $1\dfrac{5}{8}$

6. 2

7. $1\dfrac{2}{7}$

8. $\dfrac{9}{14}$

9. $8\dfrac{2}{3}$

10. $3\dfrac{12}{37}$

Decimals (pages 299–306)

A. Write in Numbers

1. 24.2	**6.** 3.003
2. 10.4	**7.** 0.0009
3. 16.29	**8.** 32.0027
4. 30.15	**9.** 0.00006
5. 0.261	**10.** 25.00085

B. Change to Fractions (reduce to lowest terms)

1. $\dfrac{5}{10} = \dfrac{1}{2}$ 　　　　**6.** $\dfrac{35}{100} = \dfrac{7}{20}$

2. $\dfrac{4}{10} = \dfrac{2}{5}$ 　　　　**7.** $\dfrac{548}{1000} = \dfrac{137}{250}$

3. $\dfrac{53}{100}$ 　　　　**8.** $\dfrac{973}{1000}$

4. $\dfrac{25}{100} = \dfrac{1}{4}$ 　　　　**9.** $\dfrac{4535}{10,000} = \dfrac{907}{2000}$

5. $\dfrac{16}{100} = \dfrac{4}{25}$ 　　　　**10.** $\dfrac{7246}{10,000} = \dfrac{3623}{5000}$

C. Change to Decimals

1. 0.3	**6.** 0.9
2. 0.2	**7.** 0.5
3. 0.4	**8.** 0.4
4. 0.8	**9.** 0.3
5. 0.8	**10.** 0.4

D. Add Decimals

1. 1.96	**6.** 174.086
2. 30.30	**7.** 89.4406
3. 15.115	**8.** 2536.74636
4. 31.095	**9.** 36.282716
5. 212.215	**10.** 247.3781

E. Subtract Decimals

1. 22.15	**6.** 0.850648
2. 382.092	**7.** 16.8914
3. 1.68	**8.** 10.7187
4. 89.1664	**9.** 768.992
5. 172.2362	**10.** 677.3118

F. Round off Decimals

1. 2.3		**6.** 15.40
2. 3.4		**7.** 3.290
3. 32.7		**8.** 291.635
4. 16.79		**9.** 782.5
5. 41.11		**10.** 2.7

G. Multiply Decimals

1. 13.04		**6.** 0.005
2. 8.15		**7.** 0.0522
3. 299.52		**8.** 0.223248
4. 107.2162		**9.** 1.638
5. 6003.46		**10.** 21.249

H. Divide Decimals

1. 40		**6.** 0.1
2. 2.8		**7.** 3
3. 2.9		**8.** 14.8
4. 4.5		**9.** 2018.2
5. 8.6		**10.** 0.1

Appendix B
Conversion Between Celsius and Fahrenheit Temperatures

Practice: Convert Temperatures (page 308)

1. 40°C	**5.** 43.3°C	**8.** 125.6°F
2. 82.4°F	**6.** 98.6°F	**9.** 37°C
3. 37.2°C	**7.** 33.3°C	**10.** 93.2°F
4. 48.2°F		

Appendix C
Measuring and Recording Fluid Balance

Calculate Fluid Balance (pages 309–310)

A. Intake: 3950 mL   **B.** Output: 2600 mL

Appendix E
Twenty-Four Hour Clock

Practice: Convert traditional to 24-hour time (page 315)

1. 1500 hours	**5.** 2130 hours	**8.** 2200 hours
2. 1000 hours	**6.** 0700 hours	**9.** 0800 hours
3. 1700 hours	**7.** 2100 hours	**10.** 1815 hours
4. 2400 hours		

Practice: Convert 24-hour time to traditional time (page 315)

1. 4:00 P.M.	**5.** 10:45 P.M.	**8.** 11:15 A.M.
2. 8:15 A.M.	**6.** 10:30 A.M.	**9.** 12 noon
3. 5:00 P.M.	**7.** 8:00 A.M.	**10.** 9:30 A.M.
4. 8:15 P.M.		

Index

License Agreement for Delmar Publishers
an International Thomson Publishing company

Educational Software/Data

You the customer, and Delmar incur certain benefits, rights, and obligations to each other when you open this package and use the software/data it contains. BE SURE YOU READ THE LICENSE AGREEMENT CARE-FULLY, SINCE BY USING THE SOFTWARE/ DATA YOU INDICATE YOU HAVE READ, UN-DERSTOOD, AND ACCEPTED THE TERMS OF THIS AGREEMENT.

Your rights:

1. You enjoy a non-exclusive license to use the en-closed software/data on a single microcomputer that is not part of a network or multi-machine system in consideration for payment of the re-quired license fee, (which may be included in the purchase price of an accompanying print compo-nent), or receipt of this software/data, and your acceptance of the terms and conditions of this agreement.

2. You own the media on which the software/data is recorded, but you acknowledge that you do not own the software/data recorded on them. You also acknowledge that the software/data is furnished "as is," and contains copyrighted and/or proprietary and confidential information of Delmar Publishers or its licensors.

3. If you do not accept the terms of this license agree-ment you may return the media within 30 days. However, you may not use the software during this period.

There are limitations on your rights:

1. You may not copy or print the software/data for any reason whatsoever, except to install it on a hard drive on a single microcomputer and to make one archival copy, unless copying or printing is ex-pressly permitted in writing or statements recorded on the diskette(s).

2. You may not revise, translate, convert, disassem-ble or otherwise reverse engineer the software/data except that you may add to or rearrange any data recorded on the media as part of the normal use of the software/data.

3. You may not sell, license, lease, rent, loan, or oth-erwise distribute or network the software/data except that you may give the software/data to a stu-dent or an instructor for use at school or, tem-porarily at home.

Should you fail to abide by the Copyright Law of the United States as it applies to this software/data your li-cense to use it will become invalid. You agree to erase or otherwise destroy the software/data immediately

after receiving note of Delmar Publishers' termina-tion of this agreement for violation of its provisions.

Delmar Publishers gives you a LIMITED WAR-RANTY covering the enclosed software/data. The LIMITED WARRANTY can be found in this product and/or the instructor's manual that accompanies it.

This license is the entire agreement between you and Delmar Publishers interpreted and enforced under New York law.

Limited Warranty

Delmar Publishers warrants to the original licensee/pur-chaser of this copy of microcomputer software/data and the media on which it is recorded that the media will be free from defects in material and workmanship for ninety (90) days from the date of original purchase. All implied warranties are limited in duration to this ninety (90) day period. THEREAFTER, ANY IMPLIED WARRANTIES, INCLUDING IMPLIED WAR-RANTIES OF MERCHANTABILITY AND FIT-NESS FOR A PARTICULAR PURPOSE ARE EX-CLUDED. THIS WARRANTY IS IN LIEU OF ALL OTHER WARRANTIES, WHETHER ORAL OR WRITTEN, EXPRESSED OR IMPLIED.

If you believe the media is defective, please return it during the ninety day period to the address shown below. A defective diskette will be replaced without charge provided that it has not been subjected to misuse or damage.

This warranty does not extend to the software or in-formation recorded on the media. The software and in-formation are provided "AS IS." Any statements made about the utility of the software or information are not to be considered as express or implied warranties. Delmar will not be liable for incidental or consequen-tial damages of any kind incurred by you, the con-sumer, or any other user.

Some states do not allow the exclusion or limitation of incidental or consequential damages, or limitations on the duration of implied warranties, so the above limi-tation or exclusion may not apply to you. This warranty gives you specific legal rights, and you may also have other rights which vary from state to state. Address all correspondence to:

Delmar Publishers
3 Columbia Circle
P.O. Box 15015
Albany, NY 12212-5015

This exciting CD-ROM is an interactive multimedia presentation that has been designed to enhance self-paced learning and provide you with a comprehensive learning package. Reduce any test anxiety you may experience by practicing at your own pace.

Features include:

- Tutorial to help you get started
- 300-word glossary
- Audio pronunciation of drug names
- Testing assessment tool with scoring capabilities
- Review questions with answers and rationales
- Practice problems with answers and rationales
- Critical thinking skills
- Color photographs
- 160 Drug labels
- Audio pronunciation of common sound-alike drug names
- Intuitive and attractive interface
- Help feature
- Toll-free technical support
- Plus Flash!™, an electronic flash card program

CD-ROM Set-up Instructions

Hardware Requirements

- 33 MHz 386 w/4MB of RAM
- Recommended 486 w/8MB of RAM
- Windows™ 3.1 or later; sound card
- VGA with 256 color display
- Double-spin CD-ROM drive
- 4MB free disc space

Installation

Before you run the installation program, check the system requirements noted above. This program will take approximately 4 megabytes of disc space.

Windows™ 3.1

To install the Clinical Calculations: A Unified Approach CD-ROM, start Windows™. Insert the disc in the CD-ROM drive. From the Program Manager, click on "File," then "Run." Type "D:\SETUP" or "E:\SETUP" and press OK. The drive letter indicated depends on the drive designated for the computers CD-ROM drive.

Windows™ 95

Insert the disc in the CD-ROM drive. Select "Start" and "Run:" Type "D:\SETUP" or "E:\SETUP" and press OK. The drive letter indicated depends on the drive designated for the computers CD-ROM drive. Installation of video playback software is not required in Windows™ 95.

Sounds in Windows™ 3.1

If sound does not play while running the Clinical Calculations: A Unified Approach CD-ROM within Windows™ 3.1, check to be sure that your sound card is set up according to the manufacturer's instructions.

The MCI-CD Audio Driver must be installed. From the Main Group in Windows™ Program Manager, open Control Panel and select the "Drivers" option. Scroll through the installed drivers list. If [MCI] CD Audio is not installed, you will need your original Windows™ installation discs to proceed. Select "Add" and select the [MCI] CD Audio driver from the list.

Technical Support

Call 1-800-824-5179 9:30 A.M. to 4:30 P.M. Eastern Standard Time *or* Fax 1-800-880-9496 24 hrs. a day

Microsoft® is a registered trademark and Windows™ and Video for Windows™ are trademarks of Microsoft Corporation. Flash!™ is a registered trademark of Delmar Publishers.